BOOKS SHOULD BE RETURNED ON OR BEFORE THE LAST DATE SHOWN
BELOW. BOOKS NOT ALREADY REQUESTED BY OTHER READERS MAY
BE RENEWED BY PERSONAL APPLICATION, BY WRITING, OR BY
TELEPHONE. TO RENEW, GIVE THE DATE DUE AND THE NUMBER ON
THE BARCODE LABEL.

FINES CHARGED FOR OVERDUE BOOKS WILL INCLUDE POSTAGE
INCURRED IN RECOVERY. DAMAGE TO, OR LOSS OF, BOOKS WILL BE
CHARGED TO THE BORROWER.

...OME

...BACK

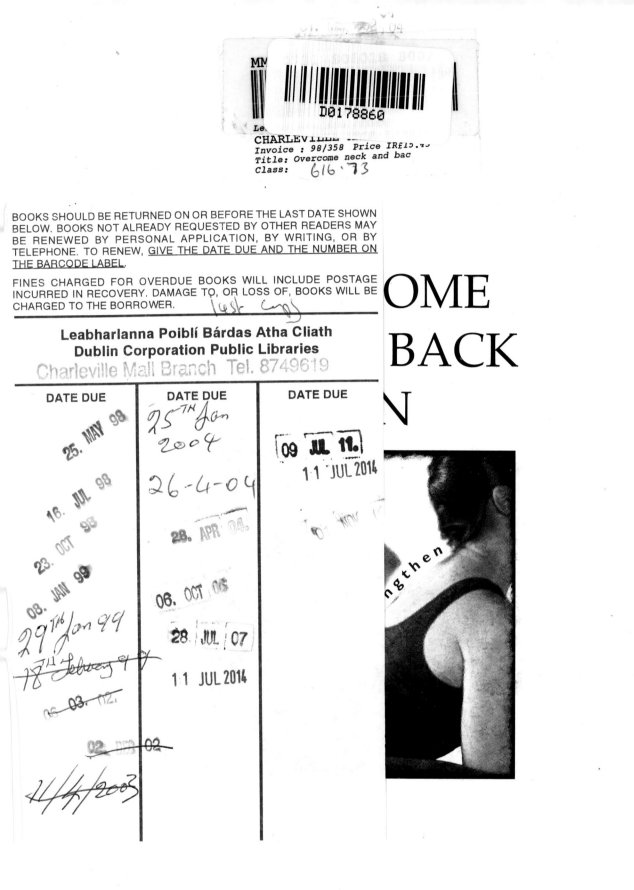

DATE DUE	DATE DUE	DATE DUE
25. MAY 98	25TH Jan 2004	09 JUL 11.
16. JUL 98	26-4-04	11 JUL 2014
23. OCT 98	28. APR 04.	
08. JAN 99	06. OCT 08	
29th Jan 99	28. JUL 07	
18th February 99	11 JUL 2014	
06. 03. 02.		
02. DEC 02		
11/4/2003		

OVERCOME

NECK & BACK

PAIN

KIT LAUGHLIN

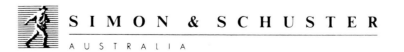
SIMON & SCHUSTER
AUSTRALIA

OVERCOME NECK & BACK PAIN

First published in 1995 by BodyPress

This revised edition published in Australia in 1996 by
Simon & Schuster Australia
20 Barcoo Street, East Roseville NSW 2069

Reprinted 1997 (three times)

Viacom International
Sydney New York London Toronto Tokyo Singapore

National Library of Australia
Cataloguing in Publication data

Laughlin, Kit, 1953 –.
    Overcome neck and back pain.

    Rev. ed.
    Bibliography.
    ISBN 0 7318 0601 8.

    1. Neck pain – Exercise therapy. 2. Backache – Exercise
    therapy. I. Title.

617.53062

Design by Jeremy Mears
Produced in Hong Kong by Bookbuilders Ltd.

To my mother and my father

ABOUT THIS BOOK...

This book is for anyone who has suffered neck or back pain, or who wishes to avoid it. It is also for anyone who seeks to develop and maintain a strong and supple spine through to old age.

There are three main elements to the approach in this book: stretching, strengthening and relaxation exercises, which are presented in an easy-to-learn format with detailed photographs and clear anatomical diagrams and explanations. The book takes you from gentle stretching exercises that help identify the problem area, to advanced exercises designed to strengthen and protect the area, and includes a special section just for athletes and those accustomed to more serious training.

For those seeking more detailed explanation, there is a separate chapter outlining causes of neck and back pain from the perspectives of different types of medicine, including an analysis of the author's approach, which may be useful for those involved in these areas.

The book is a genuinely new approach to the self-treatment of neck and back pain.

HOWEVER...

This book has been written for a wide audience, and the information is necessarily very general. It does not attempt to offer medical advice to any particular reader, each having his or her own strengths and weaknesses, which this book is not able to take into account. This book cannot be regarded as a substitute for professional medical advice or treatment, and it is recommended that you seek medical advice before commencing any exercise.

The information contained in this book is based on the author's own research, and is accurate to the best of his knowledge. However, the author does not accept any liability whatsoever for any damage arising from the information or statements contained in this book, or in connection with the use of the information.

CONTENTS

ILLUSTRATIONS

WHY THE INTEREST IN NECK AND BACK PAIN?

It seems that everyone has suffered neck or back pain at some stage. Neck or back pain affects between 60% and 85% of people. Probably you are one of these people. In one study, researchers reported that 21% of patients experienced back pain in the 14 days preceding the study. Another study reported that at least 5% of all patient visits to the doctor are due to back pain.

Tremendous costs are involved. More working hours in Australia are lost through back pain than from industrial action. Back pain accounts for half the worker's compensation payments in the United States and Australia, is the single greatest cause of lost work time in both countries, and costs $8,000 million annually in the United States. The 10% or so of patients who suffer chronic back pain account for 75% of Australia's rehabilitation and compensation payments. The social cost cannot be calculated—back pain is the most frequent cause of inactivity among people under 45 years of age.

However, patients are not the only ones to suffer. Back pain has been described as 'a wilderness across whose inhospitable terrain orthopaedic surgeons, neurosurgeons, physiotherapists and, above all, general practitioners are doomed to travel' (Littler, 1983). Most doctors believe 'there is little doubt that most cases are due to derangement of the intervertebral joint in association with 'degeneration' of the disc and arthrosis of the facet joints' (Ganora, 1984). And yet a recent article in the New York Times raises serious doubts about these claims: nearly two-thirds of a group studied had 'spinal abnormalities, including bulging or protruding discs, herniated discs, and degenerated discs'—but none of the subjects in the study had back pain (Kolata, 1994).

What is this book about?

I believe that most neck and back pain is experienced in the muscles associated with the spine. The pain is caused by excessive tension in these muscles and is the result of a variety of causes, from structural imbalances to various aspects of lifestyle. These causes can be addressed. Except for a very small percentage of neck and back pain which can be treated successfully by surgery or drug therapy, I advocate a conservative, exercise-based approach, the subject of this book.

My approach to overcoming neck and back pain has two parts. The first step is to help you identify which muscles are involved in your case and to teach you the most efficient ways to relieve this excess tension. This phase of treatment (the rehabilitation phase) is augmented by directed relaxation. The second step (the prevention phase) is to condition all of the relevant parts of the body by using more advanced stretching exercises and later, by adding specific strengthening exercises, to provide an increased measure of protection for the future. I shall present an approach to neck and back pain that is effective in practical terms and comprehensive in theoretical terms, and that will help to make sense of the apparently conflicting research on the problem.

Who should use this book?

This book is written for anyone who suffers neck or back pain, or who wishes to avoid these problems. Recovery is not quick and simple, but there are not many other options either. Unless your back or neck problem is of the kind that can be treated effectively by surgery or drug therapy (probably less than ten percent of the cases presented to general practitioners), you may have found that the range of options often seems limited to avoidance of the activity thought to be the cause and treatment of the symptoms. If treatment is successful, your back will be returned to normal; that is, to its 'pre-injury' level of function. There is no guarantee that the problem will not return. Of course, there are many practitioners who do far more than this, and my remarks are not addressed to them. My aim is to present a unified and comprehensive self-help approach. For those fortunate enough not to have such problems, the approach will strengthen your neck and back to reduce the likelihood of injury to these areas.

How this book is set out

The introduction sounds a more personal note than the following chapters. It begins with a brief history of events which led me to my current approach, including a rather lengthy stay in Japan, where I studied Shiatsu and a number of traditional exercise systems. I consider the various exercise systems from which I derived my own, the courses called *Posture & Flexibility*, and *Strength & Flexibility*, currently taught at the Australian National University. My clinic in Canberra (the Shoshin Centre) is mentioned, and I present some relevant neck and back pain case studies.

The first three chapters are the stretching and strengthening exercises; these are the nuts and bolts of my approach. Chapter one contains the basic pain-relieving and rehabilitation exercises; the first section describes exercises for the back, and the second describes exercises for the neck. Chapter two details the preventive stretching exercises. These are designed to improve and *balance* your existing flexibility, and allow you to locate your problem areas. Chapter three outlines my approach to strengthening exercise, and details a set of graded strength exercises, from a minimal set able to be done at home, through to more elaborate exercises for which some equipment is needed.

However, do not go straight to the exercises without reading the cautions *section below.* Inappropriate exercise may worsen your condition, and the nature of the problem is the best guide to selecting the exercises which are right for you.

You will get more out of the exercises if you have a reasonable working knowledge of the anatomy of the areas of interest. For this reason, useful *functional* anatomical information will be found together with the exercises. Organising the book this way means that you do not need to go backwards and forwards between the exercises and the anatomical details upon which the exercises so crucially depend. Experience has shown that the actual locus of neck or back pain tends to be the muscles associated with the spine. As each muscle has a clearly definable function, this knowledge will help you locate the particular group concerned, and guide you to the best exercise. The book has been bound so it can be left open on the floor beside you, to enable you to check your form as you practise.

Chapter four discusses the various causes of neck and back pain, from a number of medical perspectives beginning with that of western medicine. One of the reasons for so doing is that western medicine has the most detailed understanding of anatomy, and this knowledge is fundamental to my approach. Another reason is that we are familiar with the western medical perspective—it is the medicine of our culture. But to ignore the lessons of some of the other, much older, forms of medicine would be foolish indeed. Precisely because other forms of medicine are less technology-oriented, they have had to rely on the more manual techniques—knowledge our medicine feels it has largely superseded. This chapter includes a brief consideration of chiropractic and osteopathy because neck and back pain is the main concern of these practitioners. Oriental medicine and some of the 'bodywork' schools are also considered. Acute and chronic pain are treated separately, and mention made of additional contributing factors. The chapter ends with a note on the limitations of the very *idea* of cause with respect to common illnesses, which underpins my 'functional' approach.

Chapter five provides a rationale for including relaxation techniques as part of the larger approach to overcoming neck and back pain. It discusses practical stress management, outlines the current understanding of stress and its effects on the body, and ends with an easy-to-learn method for relaxation. Useful guided visualisation techniques for speeding up the healing process are included in the relaxation script.

Cautions

Before you begin, some notes of caution must be sounded. If you are undergoing some form of treatment at the moment, you must discuss the exercises presented in the book with your practitioner *before* beginning. It is a matter both of courtesy and safety—some of the exercises may be inappropriate (contraindicated in medical parlance) for your condition. Further, embarking on a course of exercises that have not been examined or approved by your practitioner may make any compensation to which you may be entitled irrecoverable. I have written this book in good faith, but I cannot be there to supervise your performance of the movements, and therefore cannot accept any responsibility for errors you make. Neither can I know the particular details of a condition you may have—this is your responsibility. *These facts necessitate the greatest caution on your part*—the fact that thousands of people have benefited from this system is no guarantee that you will. Therefore you must approach the exercises with caution, and you must monitor the effects closely.

Next, do not refer only to the photographs. You must read the sometimes lengthy descriptions that accompany them. Information vital to safety is contained in the text, along with descriptions of how to press or pull certain parts in certain ways. It is not possible to understand the exercises only by looking at the photographs.

The next caution concerns the order in which the exercises are presented. In most cases the easiest and safest versions of any movement are shown first. This is the order in which you should attempt them. The exceptions are those exercises that need to be shown in a particular form for teaching purposes—in these cases, the easier versions may follow. In either case, even if you know that you can do a more difficult version, begin with the simpler one. You can always learn something about the way your body works from doing an **easier** rather than a more difficult version of an exercise, simply because you can concentrate more on your responses to a movement rather than its complexities. Additionally, the easier versions are a useful warm-up for the later ones.

Lastly, I wish to discuss some practical cautions. You must not exercise within an hour and a half of eating. It is best to exercise in the hour before you eat the evening meal. Always go to the toilet before exercising. Wear clothing that both keeps you warm, and permits free movement. Some of the exercises require a strong towel, so have one handy. Exercise in the evenings rather than the mornings; the body is more supple then. For the first few weeks or months, I suggest that you stretch only twice a week, which may be increased to three times as you improve. The text includes specific instructions on the few exercises I recommend be done daily to relieve the body of the effects of the day's stress. More of this later.

The following caution may be self-evident, but permit me to labour a vital point. You must imitate the *form* of the exercises demonstrated, not my *performance* of them. The purpose of the precise descriptions and photographs is so that you can place yourself in the positions I have found to produce the best results. You then proceed with the stages of the movements *only until you feel the stretch I describe, and at that point you stop*. In the demonstration of the movement, I may have taken the particular limb further in the range of movement than you can, but this is immaterial. (You may well be able to stretch further than I in some exercises, too.) The *feeling* of the stretch in the right place is the sole purpose of the exercise. Please keep this in mind—most teaching of stretching exercise fails on this crucial point.

The most general, and important, caution I have saved until last. It is that you must *listen* to what your body tells you while you are doing the movements; no-one else can do this for you, not even the best teacher. Very early in your practice you must learn the essential difference between the right kind of stretch sensation and going too far. For this reason, I urge you to do too little rather than too much in the beginning—realising the difference too late will be painful, and possibly dangerous. Remember: 'Rome was not built in a day'.

The Introduction provides you with the background to the approach advocated in the book. If you prefer, you may go straight to chapter one, the rehabilitation stretching exercises, and return to the Introduction at a later time.

BACKGROUND TO THE APPROACH

In this introduction, I should like to give you some personal details, which I hope will both be interesting and give you some insight into the whys and wherefores of the methods presented in the rest of the book.

During the early 1980s, I was a television director and a struggling athlete. I trained for the 800 and 1500 metre races, the so-called 'middle distance' events. Directing the Australian Broadcasting Commission's *Nationwide* was stressful enough on its own; together with all the running training—we ran 100 miles (160 km) a week in the winter months—I now think that I was asking too much of myself. I used to hold a tremendous amount of tension in the middle back muscles. Despite physiotherapy and chiropractic treatments, the problem never really improved beyond temporary relief.

Some sort of insight occurred one day when I bent down to touch my toes after a training session. At full stretch my fingers came a few inches below my knees, and that was with my back bent like a pretzel. Someone took a photograph of me trying to do this, and it ended up on the wall at my local gym, suitably inscribed 'Rubber Man'.

The next insight occurred when I was using the calf raise machine (from the seated position a padded bar is lifted on the knees to strengthen the *soleus,* one of the two calf muscles). I placed my feet evenly on the footrest and positioned my heels level with each other. One knee contacted the support bar. The other was a full centimetre or so lower. Naturally, my first thought was that the machine was bent. I looked at it carefully, and decided that it was straight. Only then did the possibility that *I* might not be straight occur to me. Careful measurement revealed that my right leg from knee to heel was noticeably shorter than my left. I mention this only to highlight the point that we resist the notion that there might be something less than ideal in our own physical make-up. However, open-mindedness is essential if we wish to overcome our problems.

Once I had accepted the difference (in fact my right leg is shorter by about two centimetres, evenly divided between the upper and lower leg), I began to think about the effects this might have caused. I realised that years of weight training adapted my body to two major stresses—the stresses of the training itself, and the asymmetric distribution of those forces as resolved in my particular body. I began 'limber' classes at a Sydney dance studio. I soon realised that the approach adopted in these classes was not efficient for teaching adults how to become flexible. The young students were already flexible and had become flexible while they were still children. These classes were simply preparation, a warm-up, for their ballet classes later in the day. My experience there made me think about the differences between adults' and childrens' bodies, and how one might improve the standard approaches to becoming flexible.

At this time, I experimented with lifts of various thicknesses in my right shoe. The difference it made to running was immediately apparent. The shooting pains in between the shoulder blades experienced in the finishing stretches of my races all but disappeared, and on using the insert the first time, I felt more balanced walking and running.

During the late 1970s I attended yoga classes at various places around Sydney. I found the classes relatively inflexible in the sense that the approaches ranged from doctrinaire to almost militaristic. I found the 'guru mentality' oppressive, and many of the teachers had adopted the mannerisms and aphorisms of their teachers, whose words were Law. The atmosphere discouraged questions at the very time one needed assistance. I did not meet a teacher who had more than a passing acquaintance with anatomy—an aspect of western medicine unquestioned by the alternative therapies. (Since this book was first published, I have been reliably informed that much has changed since these days, and that anatomical knowledge is emphasised in contemporary yoga teaching.) I also resumed martial arts training, and did the kind of stretching usually employed in these arts during the warm-up—vigorous dynamic movements, assisted by a partner or an instructor, and all over in 15 minutes before the 'real' training began. I injured myself a number of times using this approach. On one occasion, I pulled a groin muscle that took nine or ten months to heal and was subsequently injured at another training session.

I had my thirtieth birthday in Japan. I had left television (or it had left me), and decided to go to the source for martial arts. I was dismayed to find the same *gung-ho* approach to stretching there too. I found disbelief on the part of teachers who could not accept that someone who had trained for ten years or so was not perfectly flexible. They had no real suggestions on how to *become* flexible. They had all done the usual stretching as children (usual in Japan, anyway) and consequently did not need to know how to make an adult flexible. The severe training I went through (I was a live-in student, called an *uchi deshi*) made my back even tighter. After nearly a year and a half of this life, I found myself unable to recover from a cold that alternated between a cold and the 'flu for six months. A friend had been studying a form of oriental medicine for a year or so (*shiatsu*) and, sick of being kept awake at night when I visited, he suggested that I go to see his teacher.

It was a revelation. Never have I let anyone hurt me so much. I was holding a tremendous amount of tension, and all the places he worked on, including my back, were incredibly tender to touch. I was sceptical of a treatment that consisted merely of pressing on various places. However, I started to feel better that same day, and by the time of the next treatment (a week later) the cold had gone. It was at the conclusion of the second treatment that I met a woman who would change my way of thinking about flexibility. Ms K— was a diminutive Japanese woman around 35 years old. She was introduced as the translator for the shiatsu classes foreigners attended at the centre. My teacher mentioned that I was interested in becoming more flexible. Ms K—'s way of getting to the floor involved sliding through the side splits into front splits, then lifting herself into *seiza*, the normal Japanese way of sitting, on one's feet. It was most impressive.

Ms K— and I were to do considerable work together on flexibility, and shiatsu, as I became a student. She was the sole surviving *shihan* (teacher) of an exercise method called Jikyo Jutsu. Roughly translated, this means 'self-help method'. Like *Tai Chi*, it is based on meridian theory, the practice of which is designed to 'harmonise energy flow' around the body and promote internal health, in much the same way as shiatsu. This internal health is said to be responsible for the flexibility that ensues. In other words, the acquisition of flexibility was deemed to be a side effect of health. Quite different to our western approach, I thought. The exercises themselves were an interesting mixture of dynamic stretching movements and pressure point therapy. In time I was awarded a *shodan* (a 'first degree' black belt). 'Sho' is the character for 'beginning', and unlike other parts of the world where a black belt is a pinnacle of achievement, in Japan it signifies a starting point.

Part of the learning process of shiatsu involves receiving treatment from one's teacher. I received treatment for months on a fortnightly basis, did the Jikyo Jutsu, and taught and attended yoga classes in Tokyo. After three years or so, my back felt considerably better and my flexibility was noticeably improved, particularly when I cast my mind back to the 'Rubber Man' era. All was progressing. An incident one day on my way to teaching yoga at the well-known 'Clark-Hatch' gym in Tokyo soon dispelled my complacency. While walking across the car park (thinking about something else), I inadvertently stepped off a low kerb—no more than seven or eight centimetres high—and felt a stabbing pain in my lower back. The sensation was so strong it literally took my breath away. I continued walking to the gym, and although my back did not feel 'right', I taught the class. When I returned home that evening, I stripped off and looked at myself in the full-length mirror in the bathroom. Unbelievably, my hips seemed displaced so much to one side that the normal indentation of the waist had completely disappeared on one side, compensated for by double the amount on the other. I had trouble accepting the evidence of my eyes; I could not believe what I was seeing.

The following days revealed that this distortion was going to be with me for some time. I had treatment variously from my shiatsu teacher, a well-known local chiropractor, and in desperation yet another shiatsu teacher. None altered the displacement by any extent that I could see or feel. Worse still were their claims that they had not seen any equivalent problem in all their years of practice. I was so worried by this that I travelled four hours north of Tokyo to another chiropractor, but he could not help either. Very slowly, with careful stretching over a period of seven or eight weeks, my shape returned to normal. I now think that the incident resulted from an imbalance of too much flexibility and not enough strength, my body being predisposed to injury due to my leg-length difference.

I spent considerable time thinking about the physical structures involved. One chiropractor suggested that the distortion resulted from one hip bone (ilium) moving with respect to the sacrum (in effect, driven upwards by the unexpected force of stepping off the kerb onto my shorter leg while completely relaxed). This joint, particularly in men, is normally stable and the ligaments binding the sacroiliac joints on both sides of the pelvis are extremely strong. It is possible that all the hip abduction work I had been doing (legs-apart stretching) had upset the stability of the *pubic symphysis*, thereby permitting the much more stable sacroiliac joint to move. However, because the shape of the distortion appeared simply to be an extremely exaggerated version of the normal lateral curve in my lumbar spine induced by my leg-length difference, I thought this unlikely. When my own teacher suggested that enough shiatsu treatment would even up the length of my legs, I felt that I needed to consider the problem in depth.

The apparently conflicting explanations I had been offered for the problem led me to think about standards of evidence and relationships between information produced in different frameworks. It seemed to me then (and seems so today) that there are various *kinds* of facts about the world, and that there are different expectations of reliability about these facts. 'Information' or 'facts' come bound together with indices of reliability, and these aspects together are what facts really are. In respect to my back problem, for example, it was not that one perspective was 'wrong' and another 'right'. Each perspective provided one window on the problem—a window that revealed a particular view.

These musings led me to think that, in respect to a health problem, we can conveniently divide the body into psychological and physical aspects, as western medicine ordinarily does. The physical body can be considered in terms of a spectrum, from its least-alterable to most-alterable substances, as one way of deciding how to tackle the problem. One advantage of working with the physical aspects of a body (in contrast to the psychological) is that cause and effect relationships are better known, and are often measurable. For example, we know that the nerves of the body react most quickly to stress, followed by the muscles, then ligaments and tendons, and the last to change are the hardest substances in the body—the bones and teeth. How these substances manifest their reactions to particular stresses is well known. For a problem like neck or back pain, we can affect the nerves (using the relaxation techniques), we can affect the results of stress (by using the stretching exercises), and we can strengthen the body against future stress.

This approach seems like a structural and engineering analysis, but the oriental 'umbrella' permits useful association of aspects whose precise causal relationship is not clear. The oriental perspective allows greater freedom than the western medical approach, because it is a medicine of *correlation* rather than cause—it is a system of correspondence (Porkert, 1974). I will discuss the problems of causality further in chapter four. The essence of my approach is that in multi-causal problems you direct your analysis and treatment towards the solution of the problem rather than solving the problems of causality. This approach can avoid the pitfalls of symptomatic treatment.

Shoshin Centre

In 1988 I opened the Shoshin Centre, specialising in shiatsu. One of the four main forms of oriental medicine in the modern world, shiatsu uses manual pressure on the acupuncture points for treatment, and was developed in Japan. Although I began with the intention of practising preventive medicine, I quickly realised that most patients were seeking a cure for a particular problem affecting them at the time. Although I stressed lifestyle modification and the application of specific exercises for long-term resolution of problems, most patients preferred to return at three or six-month intervals for treatment. By the end of the first year, it was clear that most of my patients wanted help with neck and back pain more than any other problem, and this pattern has continued to this day.

At any initial consultation in my clinic, I state that we should both know after a treatment or two whether my approach is likely to be effective, and stress that any exercise recommended is an integral part of treatment. It is essential to the medium and long-term success of any treatment that patients take responsibility for their problems. Most patients are agreeably surprised to be so actively involved in the outcome of the treatment. For many, it is a new experience.

Case studies from the clinic

I should like to mention the experiences of a few patients briefly, for they illustrate my method at work and the types of problems for which it might prove helpful.

The first concerns a young (21) male rower. He came to me complaining of back pain caused, he said, by lifting a rowing 'shell' out of the water. These were the only details he gave me. When I examined him, I found a marked scoliosis (lateral curvature of the upper spine), with the right shoulder carried high on the outside of a left-facing concavity. He was right-handed and, as you would expect, the development of the right side of the spine was noticeably greater than the left. He rowed on the left side of the boat so that, in addition to the uneven development caused by the scoliosis, he displayed an extra muscular development caused both by being right-handed, and the fact that the right shoulder was moving through a greater arc than the left (due to the rotation that sweep rowing adds to the extension of the basic rowing movement). Although he complained of low back pain when we first spoke, I asked him whether his middle and upper back also troubled him. As this was so, my first suggestion was for him to train on the other side of the boat once or twice a week and to report back.

Turning then to his low back pain, I performed the usual tests of functional flexibility, concentrating on a comparison of left and right. There were marked differences in all the relevant tests, but no discernible leg-length difference. I enrolled him in a beginners' stretching class, and after a couple of months he reported that the pain had gone. We then embarked on a strengthening program, and I was fascinated to see that although a nationally competitive rower, he had very poor strength in the abdominal muscles. Considering the excellent development of the upper and lower body, I considered it likely that this lack of strength was a contributing cause of his problems (just because the waist would not be capable of transmitting the strength of either the arms or legs without distortion). To address this, I developed the basis of the waist strengthening program offered in this book. After concentrating on the stretching and strengthening exercises for about eight months, he competed in the annual 'Nationals' for rowers, recording the third-highest ergometer score without a trace of back pain. Today, some three years later, there has not been any recurrence of the original problem.

The extraordinary aspect of this case was that after the Nationals, this man's doctor revealed to me that when the rower 'hurt his back' the year before while lifting the boat out of the water, he had in fact suffered a 'massive extrusion of the L5-S1 intervertebral disc, so much so that he had displayed various neurological deficits' at that time. As you will see, neurological deficits are hard evidence of nerve impingement and serious pathology. Even in the case of demonstrable pathology—of the sort often requiring surgery—the approach I advocated was successful. I realise that this is a highly unusual case and perhaps is evidence only of the superior recuperative capacities of top athletes. Nonetheless, providing one has the support of one's doctor, I urge a conservative 'wait-and-see' approach initially, followed by cautious stretching exercise, finally followed by strengthening exercises as the condition improves.

Another interesting case began with a 'phone call from a man desperate to return to work. Originally a case of acute onset back pain, the treatments he sought were not successful and the pain had become chronic over an eighteen month period. His complaint included the original back pain and referred pain down one leg. His radiographer's report noted a 'right-facing concavity of the lumbar spine' but normal joint structures and no disc abnormalities. When I tested this man, I found a leg-length difference of about 12–15 millimetres, and a commensurate pattern of flexibility. The referred pain was experienced in the longer leg. A heel insert and just three stretching exercises had this person back at his job with much reduced discomfort. He called me recently to let me know that he was still well after a year. He said that, provided he did the exercises once or twice a week, he had no problems. In his case, I believe that the original trauma (he had slipped walking down the stairway from a local-service 'plane two years before) had resulted in a muscle injury that, due to the leg-length difference, had not had a chance to recover fully. The pain he suffered appeared to be located in the *quadratus lumborum* on the side of the longer leg. Accordingly, a heel lift of five millimetres and appropriate stretching exercises were prescribed. In his example, the side-bending with legs apart stretch provided immediate relief from the back pain itself, and the groin stretch revealed one hip flexor to be very much tighter than the other. Stretching this muscle group reduced his excessive lumbar lordosis within a couple of weeks.

Of course, not all case studies document these kinds of successes. It would be remiss of me not to mention a failure or two as well, in the interests of admitting the limits of this approach. A young woman saw me about three years ago with back pain, which her doctor had said was caused by a partial extrusion of the *nucleus pulposus*, the gelatinous core of the intervertebral disc. He advised surgery, but because her symptoms had not progressed to the stage of displaying neurological deficits, she felt that a conservative, exercise-based approach would be worth trying. I treated her a couple of times with shiatsu and, although we identified the exercises that gave her relief at the time and whose effects lasted a few days or so, eventually the pain became so intense that she had to have the operation. About eight months was needed for her to determine the outcome of the operation, which was successful. She continues to do the exercises from time to time, and reports that her back has much improved.

The final case study I saved until last because in one sense it is the most dramatic. A small middle-aged woman came to me complaining of 'excruciating' back pain. She had not responded to any treatment (and she seemed to have tried them all). Back pain had plagued her for 14 years. Her job entailed travelling extensively, and she felt that the many hours she spent in the car each week were contributing to her problem. She had bought an expensive after-market seat for her car, featuring an adjustable lumbar roll and firm side supports. The pain had not improved with this modification, but neither had it worsened over the previous year. The pain was so intense at night that her physical relationship with her husband was non-existent. Needless to say, both were strongly affected by the illness. I began with a leg-length test which revealed a small (few millimetres) difference. Hip flexion and hamstring flexibility were within normal limits and not significantly dissimilar, I thought. When I tested her for hip flexor (*iliopsoas*) tightness, quite a different picture emerged. One hip flexor was normal. Coincidentally, I had begun this test sequence with this hip. After I tested the other, which was so tight that the leg would not move past the mid-line of the body before doing a C–R stretch, she stood up next to the bench she was using for support. She had a very peculiar look on her face—fear mixed with shock. I asked her what was wrong. She replied that this instant in time was the *first time in 14 years* that her back was not 'killing' her. This state of affairs continues to this day, and she calls me every six months or so to tell me of her progress.

I know that this particular example may appear to border on the unbelievable, even miraculous. I could not believe it myself at the time, and months after the consultation I was sure that any day I would receive a 'phone call from her to say that her old problem had returned. I can only surmise that some fibres of the hip flexor group were extraordinarily tight and, in addition to their contribution to excessive lumbar lordosis, were causing the rotation of one vertebra with respect to its neighbours, and hence the pain. It is also likely that the enforced flexion of the hip joint (brought about by all those years spent in a car) may have contributed significantly to this aspect of the problem.

Posture & Flexibility *at the Australian National University*

When I returned from Japan and enrolled at the ANU, I decided to start an exercise class. My main motive was to ensure that I did enough stretching exercise myself each week. From one class per week in 1987, the course (named *Posture & Flexibility*) has grown to 15 classes per week in 1995. I have taught the five other teachers myself, and they come from diverse backgrounds. Jennifer teaches in high school and edits books. Petra is completing a PhD in biochemistry. Mark has only recently returned from fieldwork in Indonesia for his PhD in linguistics. My brother, Dr Greg Laughlin, is a senior public servant. Carol is researching a PhD in cell biology. All attend the weekly advanced class, where information is shared and new techniques tested.

The exercise forms that have strongly influenced my present work are yoga (Hatha Yoga, and more particularly the Iyengar style) and two traditional Japanese forms, (Makko Hoo and Jikyo Jutsu). None is complete, in my opinion, and I have taken liberally from all three. Where I have identified a significant lack in all three forms (for example, in specific neck exercises), I have relied on my anatomical understanding to develop an appropriate movement. Recognising that these traditional exercise forms have objectives other than the acquisition of flexibility, I have taken from any relevant form (including dance and gymnastics) solely on the basis of furthering the goal of becoming more flexible. In this way, the goal became a *de facto* framework for relating forms which technically or historically were unrelated and whose traditional adherents (as often as not) would not like to see related. All exercises presented have been tested on hundreds, if not thousands, of students.

Very early in my attempts to formulate an approach to stretching exercise, I realised that the conventional approaches to *teaching* exercise also had serious shortcomings. As mentioned earlier, of all the exercise forms I've experienced, yoga is closest to being complete in its stretching and strengthening effects but approaches to teaching it vary from insufficiently precise to doctrinaire. I also found that some of the recommendations for poses (like the lotus) made in the most reputable of textbooks are potentially dangerous, or simply wrong when considered from an anatomical perspective. Here I am not speaking of the putative effects of a pose (which often defy explanation in the scientific framework). I am talking of suggestions like the need to 'endure excruciating pain in the knees' when practising the lotus pose. The point here is that this kind of pain will only be felt if the hip joint has insufficient external rotation to permit the movement. My view is that a number of partial poses that foster this capacity in the hip joints should be used before attempting the pose, because the knees are best not used in the strongly flexed position to generate rotational forces in the hip. This is because there is a real danger of over-stretching the knee ligaments, which are maximally exposed in this position, and much of the strength of the knee in daily life derives from ligament strength.

After teaching stretching exercise for more than ten years, I suppose the most obvious conclusion I have reached is that age is no barrier to improvement. The older student usually progresses at a slower rate than a younger one, but the difference is nowhere as great as one might expect. I have also noticed that improvement is somewhat slower in the initial weeks and months of a new stretching routine than are the results of a comparable amount of time spent on strength or aerobic training. However, improvement and its consequent effects are *relative*. Any improvement in flexibility—no matter how small in absolute terms—is experienced as a major positive event by the person concerned. Even in the most stubborn case, the absolute improvement in a particular aspect of flexibility is about 10% in a year, and the sensations of daily life are changed significantly to the person enjoying this improvement on a daily basis.

Feedback from many students over the years permits me to make some concluding remarks about the relation of practice and the outcomes of illness or injury. Students report a range of benefits. When pressed for detail, they may reply that odd random aches or pains have disappeared. Some say that movement in daily life has taken on a quality of pleasure that was not previously present. However, others have been far more specific about effects. Many people come to the classes because of the kinds of neck or back pain rife among academics and students, so that the next most commonly heard remark is that the original complaint is much improved or 'cured' completely. This is also true (although to a lesser extent, admittedly) for more insidious complaints such as repetitive strain injury, or occupational overuse syndrome, where the neck and shoulder exercises have proved beneficial in the majority of cases. It should be noted that in these kinds of illnesses lifestyle modification is usually required. As most academics and students are unable or unwilling to do this for various reasons, the exercise classes are often used as a means of coping with the problem.

Contact address and email

I am very interested in people's experiences of using the approaches detailed in the book. To that end, I have provided my work address for correspondence. Any suggestions or criticism will be considered and incorporated with acknowledgment in future editions.

Kit Laughlin
LPO Box 159
Australian National University
Canberra, ACT 2601
AUSTRALIA

email: kit.laughlin@anu.edu.au

CHAPTER ONE

REHABILITATION STRETCHING EXERCISES

We all know what stretching a muscle feels like. Everyone stretches some part of his or her body every day, even if this is only some mostly instinctive movement done while thinking about something else. What I want to do in this section is try to be more explicit about ways of thinking about stretching, and to discuss an approach which will help you to stretch more effectively.

Limits

Think about stretching for a moment. What does it mean? For most people it means moving some part of the body in a particular direction until it won't move any further. Moreover, this is accompanied by certain sensations—sometimes pleasant, and sometimes not. What stops you stretching beyond a certain point? One constraint is structural: if you are stretching your arm across (in front of) the body at shoulder height for example, no matter how flexible you are you will not be able to stretch past the point where the arm meets the front of your neck. Similarly, once the heel is against the bottom, the knee joint will close no further. However, these structural limitations are not usually the limits you have in mind when you feel you cannot stretch any further.

Another constraint is often called the 'stretch reflex'. When a muscle is stretched past a certain point, stretch receptors located in particular muscle fibres send signals to surrounding muscle fibres and cause them to contract, with the result that further elongation of the whole muscle stops. It is probably the contraction of the muscle fibres in their maximally-lengthened state that causes the sensation you feel when stretching, and that will become pain if you go beyond this point. Some anatomists believe that the main function of this reflex is to protect the associated joint from being over-stretched. Specifically, they mean that the ligamentous and bony integrity of any joint has limits constrained by its particular arrangements, and they infer that one of the functions of the stretch reflex is to protect this integrity. These mechanisms help us to avoid serious injury.

Although this protective function may be useful in the normally-flexible individual, for most adults this stretch reflex restricts further movement long before the safety of the joint is threatened. The range of available movement decreases with age, and I believe that a stretch reflex being triggered inappropriately early in a joint's range of movement is responsible for much of this loss of flexibility, and much of the muscle tension and accompanying pain experienced in daily life. How might this inappropriate reflex develop?

The answer lies in an extremely complex relationship between the central nervous system and the length and tension of the muscles it governs. Repeated patterns of stimulation form the stretch reflexes. Lifestyle patterns alter as we mature, usually becoming increasingly sedentary. Activities that form these reflexes in their youthful patterns are reduced, and body weight usually increases. These tendencies reinforce each other; and the stretch reflexes reflect these changes. In most people there are no significant physiological constraints to prevent the retention of the flexibility patterns of youth. It is merely that we change our patterns of use as we age and our reflex patterns change to reflect these changes. Physiologically, the most-often repeated or strongest patterns of stimuli are remembered best by the body. In sport, this fact forms the basis of most training: that is, repetition leads to enhanced performance. The unfortunate fact of modern life is that the most strongly reinforced patterns of most people's lives do not enhance performance in any way at all.

Another limitation to stretching is the nature of the material being stretched. Tendons and ligaments have very limited extensibility—muscles are the things we stretch. Most muscles can contract to somewhere between 50% and 70% of their normal resting length, and be stretched to about 130%. Stretching beyond this exceeds the elastic limit of the muscle fibres and will cause changes which may not be reversible in the short term. Injury results, and the muscles and associated structures need time to return to normal. This brief account does not consider the differences in forces and effects that muscles experience under fast and slow stretching regimens. The extent to which these differences are pertinent to neck and back pain will be considered below. Before we begin the exercises, let us briefly consider the different methods we may employ to become more flexible. There are two types of stretching: static stretching, which is most commonly recommended, and ballistic (or dynamic) stretching.

Static stretching

In static stretching, a limb is moved into the stretch position and held statically (without movement), usually for a minimum time of somewhere between 10 and 30 seconds. It is often suggested that a number of repetitions of the static stretch be performed. Reasons given to support recommendations for static stretching are that it is safe, and, if done carefully, does not tend to aggravate any existing injuries.

The disadvantages of this conservative approach are that, in the untrained individual, the end point of the stretched position is difficult to determine. By this I mean that it is hard for a beginner to distinguish between the point at which stretching occurs and the further point at which injury may occur. If someone has a problem in a particular area, there is a very natural tendency to hold and protect the area to avoid stretching sensitive tissues. Frequently, moving the body into a position of stretch will elicit the very pain you are trying to remedy.

The 'end-point' problem and the tendency towards protecting a sore area have two consequences: either you do not stretch far enough—and hence you will not improve—or you will not acquire an enhanced sensitivity to the region of movement which exists between stretch and injury. I call this the 'stretch window'. How this window may be opened is dealt with below.

Ballistic stretching

In ballistic stretching, stretching is achieved by momentum, exemplified by kicking as high as possible to the side or the front, as in football or the dance known as the 'cancan'. The disadvantages of this approach are well known: the risk of injury through momentary over-stretching can be high, depending on the speed and power employed. This sort of movement in sporting activities is the most frequent cause of shoulder and hamstring injuries, because the end-point of the movement is so hard to control if significant momentum is employed, and when passions are running high we ignore the warning signs.

In any method of stretching, by definition, we are moving part of the body beyond its normal active range of movement. Using momentum to stretch results in less active control for two reasons. One is that the mechanisms that sense position and stretch are less sensitive outside the normal range of movement and, also, are less sensitive at speed. The other is that, once outside the normal range of movement, one's capacity to exert muscular force drops markedly, so that even if you suddenly feel that you are going too far, you may not be able to stop yourself. For these reasons, with exceptions noted below, I do not recommend ballistic stretching as a method for becoming more flexible.

The Posture & Flexibility *approach to stretching*

This is the name given to my method for improving flexibility and awareness. *Posture & Flexibility* comprises three elements:

(i) a *contract–relax* approach to increase flexibility, within a structure of (ii) *partial poses*, which may be (iii) *partner-based*. I shall address the elements in turn, beginning with a brief history of the 'contract–relax' technique, drawn from proprioceptive neuromuscular facilitation (PNF).

(i) *Contract–relax (C–R)*

PNF is a detailed set of patterns for re-educating the neuromuscular responses. PNF was developed at the Kabat-Kaiser Institute during the late 1940s in the United States. What is sometimes called 'PNF stretching' today is a tiny fragment of a much larger set of techniques that rely on complex patterns of movement designed to re-educate the movements of people with cerebral or spinal injuries. The description of what is called the contract-relax (C–R) technique, one of three stretching techniques in the original textbook (and what most people mean when they use the term PNF stretching), is but a short paragraph on page 98 (Knott & Voss, 1968). I have taken this C–R fragment from the original PNF system and refined it over the past 15 years, and feel confident that I can offer it now as part of a fully developed method for stretching.

At its most basic, the C–R approach we use means moving the limb into a gently-stretched position, and holding it there for a short time (generally 10 to 30 seconds) until you relax and become accustomed to the feeling of being in this position. Then you *contract*—this means that you will push (or pull) the limb back *in the opposite direction to the movement used to get into the stretch position*, for somewhere between six to ten seconds; then you stop pushing. The final part of the approach requires you to restretch the same muscles (as a separate action); the new position is then held, from ten seconds to about a minute. The three parts make up one iteration of the C–R approach. In certain instances, this may be repeated, up to a maximum of three times. We have found that there is no significant improvement with further iterations in any particular stretching session.

One advantage of using the C–R approach to stretching is that it develops strength at the extremes of any range of movement. This is because the contractions increase strength through the isometric principles, covered in chapter three. Thus, not only do you become more flexible, you become stronger as well, especially in the extreme ranges of movements that are left unaltered by conventional approaches to strength or flexibility training.

The original PNF textbook does not specify how much effort to use in the contraction phase. As the techniques were developed for rehabilitation, we may assume that, in general, the therapists were dealing with relatively weak patients. When we are using the C–R technique, how hard should we contract the muscles? Experimenting with willing students and patients over the years has resulted in the following suggestions.

Presuming that you have had neck or back pain, *always* err on the side of not pushing or pulling hard enough when first trying the method, for two reasons. Assuming that we are using the C–R approach to stretch a sore area, the first consideration is that we wish to avoid over-stressing the very muscles we believe to be responsible for the pain. The second is that by being careful and 'listening' to the body's responses to a new demand, we are in a position to modify the demand as necessary.

The best way to determine how much effort to use is to push back slowly (over a few seconds) against the resistance until you can actually *feel* the muscle the particular exercise is designed to stretch. Aim to contract with only 20-30% of your maximum effort. In the beginning, we want to open the stretch window to a point between the kind of stretch sensation we judge as desirable, and what we judge is too much and that could be injurious or painful. This requires a deal of sensitivity, and people who have been in pain for a long time have lost much of the ability to make such judgements. However, work slowly and sensitively and you will be working safely. *Err on the side of pushing too little rather than too much.* We are trying to re-educate the body into being more supple—we are not trying to force it into being more supple.

As you become accustomed to working with your body, you may increase the effort expended in the contraction phase. Do this either by contracting more forcefully or by holding the contraction for a longer period. In the case of the hamstring muscles for example, in time you may find that contractions of 10 to 20 seconds give the best results. With longer contractions, increase the effort *slowly* over five to ten seconds until you reach the desired maximum. Do not contract with more than about half the available effort as we have found this will not increase the stretch effect and the extra effort will leave you feeling more sore the next day. The chance of injuring the back muscles (which have to do increased work to support the stretching position of the trunk as you contract the leg muscles more) also increases beyond this point. However, with the muscles of the neck, which are much smaller and shorter than the muscles of the leg, often only a brief contraction (of a few seconds) will be sufficient to have the desired effect. Work slowly and cautiously, and soon you will find the right contraction force for each muscle group.

To summarise, I do not recommend the ballistic approach as the first choice to increase flexibility because of the inherent danger. Static stretching (exemplified by yoga) is effective. However, it is relatively inefficient in terms of results gained for time spent, has no specific strengthening component at the end of the range of movement, and lacks the capacity to immediately reduce tension in unusually tight muscles.

The C–R approach has a number of important advantages over the static and dynamic approaches. Because you are required to perform an isometric contraction, the muscles involved become stronger at the point in the range where they are usually weak (relative to their strength in the normal range). The action of doing work in the extended position also

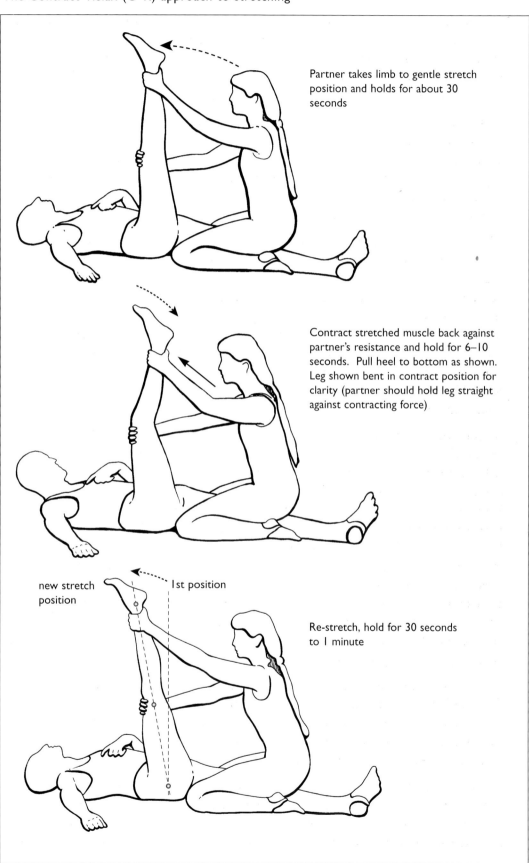

Partner takes limb to gentle stretch position and holds for about 30 seconds

Contract stretched muscle back against partner's resistance and hold for 6–10 seconds. Pull heel to bottom as shown. Leg shown bent in contract position for clarity (partner should hold leg straight against contracting force)

new stretch position

1st position

Re-stretch, hold for 30 seconds to 1 minute

increases your awareness of the stretching sensation, in effect widening the window between stretching and injuring.

Finally, your flexibility improves markedly as you use the technique; this is due to the stretch reflex being deactivated momentarily due to the activation of *Golgi organs* located at the junction of muscles and tendons whose action is to reduce the contractions in the fibres being stretched, and also perhaps due to the release of 'trigger points' in such muscles (Travell & Simons, 1983, vol. 1, p.89). But this level of detail is unnecessary here—we only need to know that there is a sound set of reasons underlying the approach.

(ii) *Partial poses*

The second element in my *Posture & Flexibility* approach is that complex movements or whole poses (from yoga, gymnastics, or dance) are broken down into an elemental vocabulary of what I call 'functional units of flexibility'. I do this to isolate a student's problem areas, and for teaching convenience. These functional units are logical elements, initially based around individual joints, progressing to multiple joints with complex movements as the student improves. Thus, a movement that requires flexibility in a number of areas simultaneously (for example, a forward bend) is broken down into calf muscle stretches, a couple of different hamstring muscle stretches, a hip stretch, a lower back stretch, and so on. Each stretch is done in turn and finally the whole movement is performed for its holistic benefits.

Focusing on specific areas of the body, accompanied by a simplified description of the anatomy involved, helps the student to visualise and feel the parts concerned and how they are integrated into the whole body. Any increase in awareness of these essential aspects aids improvement. Although the goal is to acquire whole-body suppleness, the initial focus is on improving those problem areas located by the partial poses—different for each student. This approach yields the quickest overall improvement. A tight area, even if quite small, profoundly limits more complex positions. Attention to these areas accelerates the acquisition of whole poses. In the class situation, breaking the poses down into smaller parts has the additional advantage that all students can do some of the parts, at least, which improves their confidence greatly.

(iii) *Partner-based*

The third element of the *Posture & Flexibility* approach is partner stretching. The most important advantage of using a partner in your stretching is that you do not need to supply the effort to hold yourself in any particular position. This means that you can relax in the position and attend to your breathing far more easily. Being supported by a partner means that when doing the pushing-back (contraction) part of the exercise, you can concentrate your attention in that particular muscle. The partner can keep a close eye on the *form* of the exercise—*the* crucial aspect.

We must not ignore the psychological aspects either. Doing stretching exercise with another provides support, regularity in practice, and encouragement when needed. Some authors warn of the danger of being stretched by another, but this potential problem has been largely overcome in my system, and will be covered in detail in the exercises below.

Choose someone close to your size and weight, and someone with whom you can communicate well. Your partner needs to be sensible and sensitive.

How to breathe

A final point concerns breathing during the stretching process. Contracting the muscles as an aid to stretching is hard work, and naturally your breathing rate will increase during this phase. For this reason, the direction 'to take a deep breath in before stretching' is doubly significant, for not only does it signal to the body that you are about to stretch, but breathing deeply will help your breathing and pulse rates to return to normal much more quickly. Changing your breathing patterns during the different phases of the stretching process also helps the body and the mind learn the essential *relaxation* aspect. Electromyograph studies have shown that tension increases slightly in all the muscles in the body each time you breath in, and reduces slightly each time you breath out. By focusing you attention on a breath out each time you stretch, you will enhance this natural physiological action. You cannot force muscles to relax and you cannot force them to stretch. You can however *teach* them how to behave more as you wish, and the C–R method combined with focus on breathing is the best I know for this. Accordingly, before you begin the final relaxing, stretching phase of any exercise, you should take a deep breath and make the stretching effort as you breathe out. In time, becoming conscious of breathing in and out provides a focus for more advanced techniques, covered in chapter five.

The final point to make at this stage about breathing is to note that breathing in particular ways can help the *form* of a pose too. For example, breathing in will help you straighten your back, and the directions for some exercises will ask you to 'lift the chest'. Breathing in at this time makes this direction easier to follow. On other occasions, the directions may ask you to breathe *out* as you get into the position. Usually this will be to empty the lungs momentarily to facilitate bending forward or twisting. Please pay close attention to these suggestions.

Benefits of warmth

The body is more supple when warm. We can use this knowledge to help us stretch. If the body is particularly stiff, have a hot bath before commencing the workout. Research in Germany in the 1960s indicated that the flexibility of any joint was increased 15–20% if the core temperature of the muscles was raised one to two degrees Centigrade. This is easily achieved by soaking in a hot bath. A bath is far more effective than a shower for this purpose because the hot water is in constant, relatively still, contact with the body and this facilitates heat transfer. Afterwards, dress in clothes that permit free movement but retain the heat (for example, cotton tracksuit pants and top).

Why photographs?

The last point I wish to make before we begin is that I have chosen to demonstrate the exercises myself with Jennifer, and with photographs, for two reasons. Most recent books on stretching exercises use line drawings to represent the recommended positions. This is unsatisfactory because a drawing can be made to show any position—hence one does not derive any sense of confidence from a drawing. A photograph conveys the shape and form of a position, but it does a lot more besides. You can see many fine details, such as the position of hands and feet, the precise shape of the back, and so on. There is the reassurance that the exercise really is possible, and that the person writing the book does the exercise too.

Please examine the photographs and the accompanying text carefully before attempting any exercise, *and follow the text and order of the exercises as they are presented*. Important information is included with each of the exercises, so please read the description in full while referring to the accompanying photographs before attempting them. *Do not rely on the photographs alone.*

Movement of arms and legs in the coronal plane

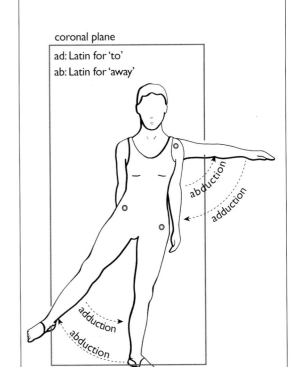

Movement of legs in the sagittal plane

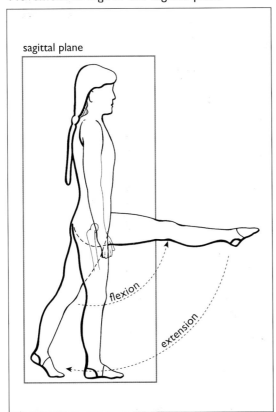

Movement of arms in the sagittal plane

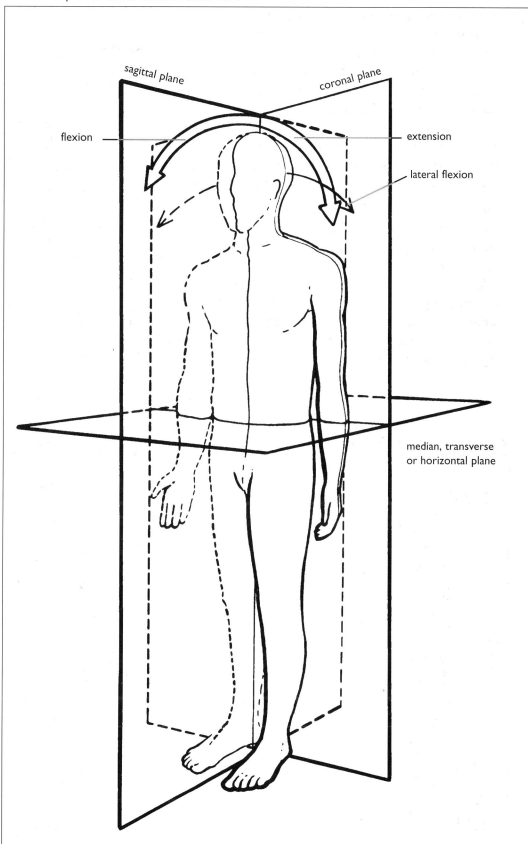

sagittal plane

coronal plane

flexion

extension

lateral flexion

median, transverse
or horizontal plane

BACK STRETCHING EXERCISES (REHABILITATION PHASE)

1. Lower back, using a chair

Let us imagine that your back is sore at this very moment. Probably the last thing you want to do is move it at all. Perhaps the usual stretching exercises do not make you feel secure—you feel too vulnerable moving into extended positions, and you feel that you may hurt yourself getting out of the position. If so, this first exercise is for you: it is designed to give a gentle stretch to the entire lower back region.

The exercise is done with the support of your arms at all times, so if you feel you are going too far you can move yourself back to the starting position by arm strength alone, thereby avoiding any additional stress on the lower back. You are in control at all times. You will need a non-sliding chair that is strong enough to support your weight, preferably without arms, and a support on the floor between your feet. This may be a strong box, a couple of large thick books, a footstool or the like. Ensure that you read all directions for the exercise, including how to get out of the final position, before attempting it.

Look at the first photograph. Here, the exercise is performed without using a support. If you think that you may not be able to bend forward to the extent of placing the fingertips on the floor, place a suitable support of some kind between your feet on the floor. Sit on the forward edge of the chair, with your weight evenly placed on both bottom bones, and with your feet placed squarely and securely on the floor slightly in front of the knees. Support the weight of the upper body with the hands on the knees, as shown. The back muscles should be *completely relaxed*, and all weight resting on the arms. Slowly (take a few seconds) let the chin go as far forward in the direction of the chest as is comfortable. This instruction is to initiate a forward bend in the upper back, and to initiate a stretch in the spinal cord. Leaning on the arms, let both arms bend slowly, allowing the body to incline forwards from the waist. (A technical note here. When doing this exercise correctly, both the spine and the hip joints will be involved; this occurs any

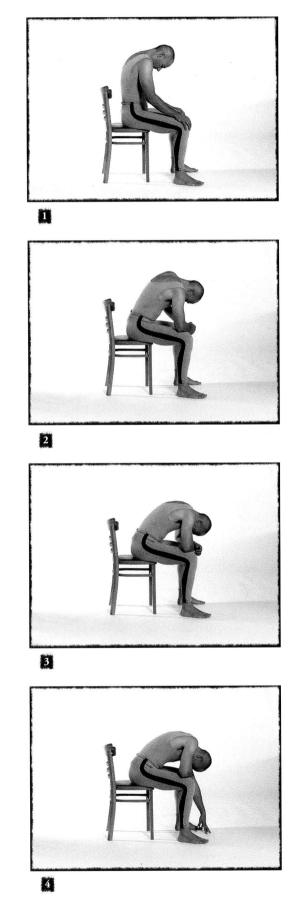

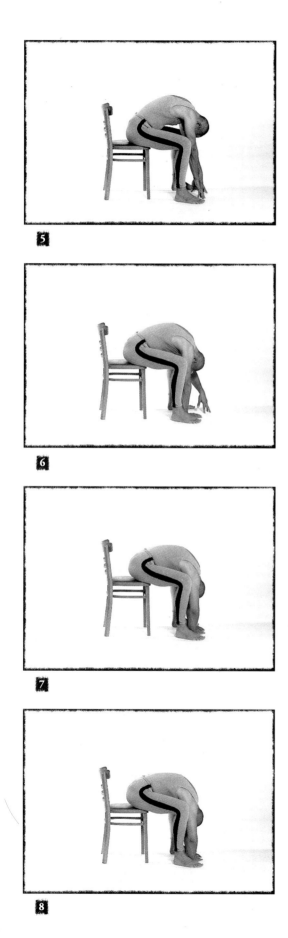

5

6

7

8

time the body moves forward between the legs.) At this time, your breathing should be completely natural—do not hold your breath for any reason. Although it may be natural to do so (perhaps in anticipation of pain or because of the newness of the movement) please resist this temptation.

Caution: if at any time you feel that you must return to the beginning position, use your arms to do so. Do not pull yourself back to the starting position with the muscles you are trying to stretch, the back muscles.

When sufficiently forward, take all your weight on one arm *without letting the body rotate*, and bend the other elbow. Now let the first arm bend and support all your weight on the elbow of the second arm. Bend the first arm now, and place it on the other leg; now you are supporting your weight evenly on both elbows. Rest for a while. Notice that although you are probably already stretching the lower back a little at this stage, because you are taking the weight on your arms, there is little or no pain.

Now we begin the real stretch. If you feel comfortable in this position, support your weight again on one elbow, and reach down to the floor with the fingertips of the other arm. If the floor looks as though it is too far away, rest this hand on the support. Taking your weight on this hand, bring the other down from your leg and rest on both hands now. Again breathe normally, perhaps with the emphasis on slightly deeper breaths than normal, but at an unhurried, unstressed rate. Take stock of what you feel—you should feel a pleasant stretching feeling in the lower back, but not pain.

Keeping your hands on either the support or the floor (whichever you are comfortable with) *very* slowly and gently unweight your arms until you feel a mild stretch in the lower back. You may well *not* need to lift the hands from the floor to achieve a sufficient degree of stretch. Let me stress the point: you must be careful, and move slowly—only you can know how far is enough. *Always* err on the side of caution. Stay in the final position for a minimum of ten breaths in and out. Do not hurry your breathing. Even though the position may feel awkward, try to breathe normally.

To return to the start position, lift the head up until you are looking forward, rest on one hand, and place the other in a support position on your leg. *Breathe in, take all your weight on this arm, bring the other into a similar support position, and lift yourself back to the original sitting position with both arms.* Now let the breath out, and relax there for a moment.

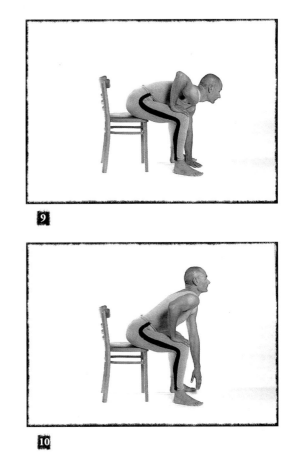

This is the first exercise, and may be done whenever the lower back feels tight, even in the office. In addition to the stretch in the lower back, you may also feel a stretch in the muscles at the back of, and inside, the legs, and the bottom muscles. All the muscles on either side of the spine, and from the top of the hips to the lower back, can be stretched using this exercise. Refer to the diagram for details of the muscles involved.

As an aside, anthropologists have noted that indigenous peoples suffer a low incidence of back pain compared with the peoples of the developed world. Of the many different aspects of their lifestyles, one aspect worth noting is that the usual way of holding discussions in these countries is to squat with the heels on the ground, rather than standing around as we do. The squatting action is a good stretch for the muscles stretched in exercise 1 and the ankles (see also exercises 28 and 29), and you may care to try it yourself. If your ankles are insufficiently flexible to allow you to balance in the position with your heels on the floor, try holding onto something secure in front of you as you bend the legs. Breath normally once in the squat position. To increase the stretch in the lower back, you may incline the body forwards from the squat position.

Muscles stretched in exercise 1

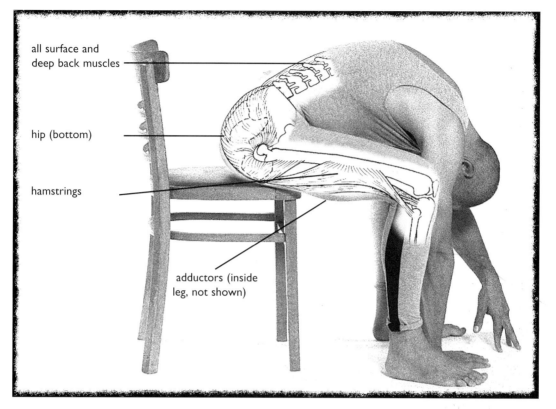

all surface and
deep back muscles

hip (bottom)

hamstrings

adductors (inside
leg, not shown)

2. Lateral flexion, using a chair and wall

So far, we have stretched mainly the muscles on either side of the spine. The next exercise emphasises the muscles that run from the top of the hip bones to the spine, and the side muscles of the waist. The final part of the movement, which involves a mild rotation of the shoulders with respect to the hips, moves this latter stretch from the side of the waist to the muscles closer to the spine itself. The exercise also uses the chair but with one side of the chair placed next to a wall. Make sure that the chair will not slide sideways away from the wall.

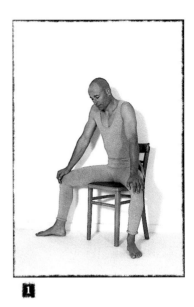

1

Lean forward onto one elbow, as shown. This time, keep the head in line with the shoulders. If your back is tender, let yourself down into this position by using the other hand, as for the previous exercise. Once supporting your weight on one elbow, lean all your weight onto it, and roll the opposite shoulder backwards until it is vertically over the shoulder on whose elbow you are leaning, or as close as you can come to this position. You can press back against the wall to help you get into the first position. Feel the stretch in the side of the waist. Still leaning on the elbow, raise the free arm and reach out in the direction of the leg you are leaning over, as shown. You can control the stretch either by the degree of reaching with the top arm, or by how much the lower arm lets the body lean to the side. You can increase the stretch by moving the supporting elbow further towards the knee, and transferring more of your weight to it. Doing this will increase the stretch in the side of the waist. Make sure that you are safely supported at all times.

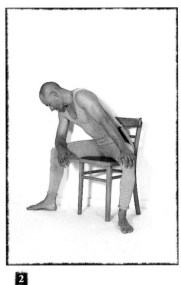

2

It may be that you feel insufficient stretch in the desired place if supported on the elbow in the manner described. If this is so, you may make the starting position a stronger stretch than outlined above by resting your body's weight on the back of your arm instead of the elbow. Alternatively, you may rest the hand on a support placed on the floor next to the ankle of the leg you intend leaning over. The support should be of a height which gives you just sufficient stretch. In the strongest version, the hand may be placed directly on the floor—this will be the maximum stretch effect position (see photograph 9 opposite page). All other instructions will be the same. Do not try these more extreme versions if the first version outlined above is effective. In most exercises, the proportions of one's body determines the strength of the effect.

Assuming that you are in one of the positions outlined, to move the stretch closer into the spine at the same time as maintaining

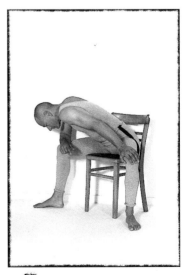

3

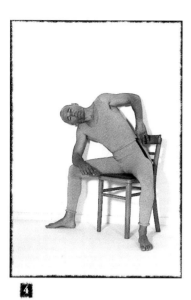

4

(or even increasing, if this feels safe) the sideways stretch, very slowly roll the top shoulder forwards in small increments. As you do this, you will feel the stretch move from the side of the waist to the muscles closer to the spine. When you have stretched sufficiently (but certainly no less than 30 seconds or so) support your weight on the elbow on your knee, return the top hand to its starting position (a similar position on the other knee), carefully transfer your weight to your hands, and use the arms to return to the starting position.

Repeat for the other side. Take particular notice of whether one side of the body is more flexible than the other. If this is the case, next time you stretch begin with the tighter side, then stretch the looser side, and re-stretch the tighter side. *Make this a general rule for all exercises that permit comparison of right and left.*

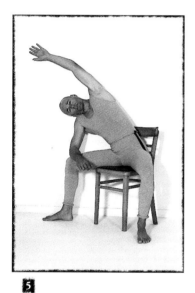

5

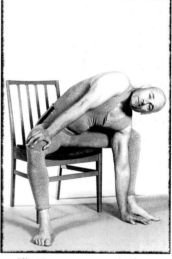

9 The strongest version

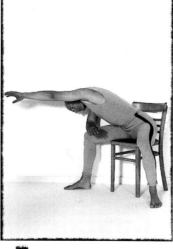

6

7

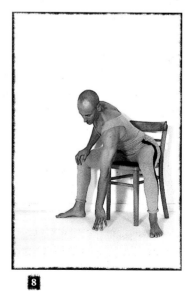

8

3. Knee to chest and rotation

The third exercise is done on the floor, preferably carpeted or on a thin foam mattress. Stretching on a bed is not suitable because the surface does not usually provide sufficient support. Lie on your back. If lying on your back in this position is painful, try getting into it this way. Lower yourself into the lying position, but keep both knees bent (flexed). Use your arms (by holding onto the knees for additional support if necessary). Clasp one knee to the chest (refer to the photographs). When secure, lower the other leg until the back of it is on the floor. Getting into the start position this way avoids arching (or, technically speaking, hyperextending) the lower back. Clasping one knee to the chest maintains a little forward curve in the lumbar spine and this will avoid the pain often associated with lying in a face-up position.

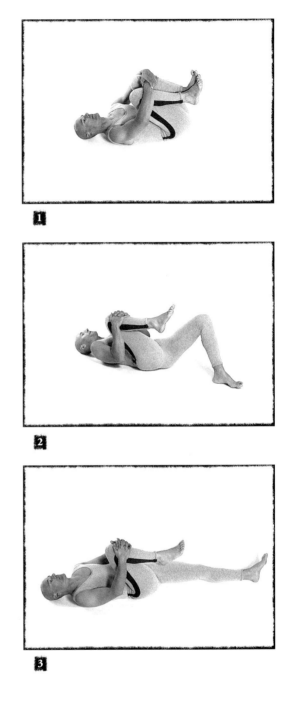

You are now ready to begin the exercise. Bring the knee to the chest. If you feel an uncomfortable pinching sensation in the groin of the bent leg, check to see whether overly-tight material around the top of the leg is the cause. If loosening the cloth does not remove the irritation, let the leg go away from the chest until arm's length, and fall further to the outside line of the body. Then bring the knee back to the body again, but this time in line with the armpit. Some people trap the tendons and muscles of the hip flexors when they pull the knee straight back to the chest. Bringing the knee into roughly the same position, but from the side, usually avoids this problem.

Now, gently pull the knee into the chest (or armpit) using both hands as shown. You may feel the stretch variously from behind the leg (top part of the hamstring muscle) to inside the leg (the adductors), and you may also feel the stretch in the bottom muscles on the bent-leg side.

After holding the stretch for about ten breaths, let the leg go to arm's length. Hold the outside of the thigh with the hand of the opposite shoulder, as shown. Roll the leg across the body. As soon as it passes over the vertical centreline of the body, take some weight on the bottom leg, *and shift the bottom hip across in the opposite direction.* This ensures that the spine, as seen from above, remains straight. Most floor rotation exercises do not include

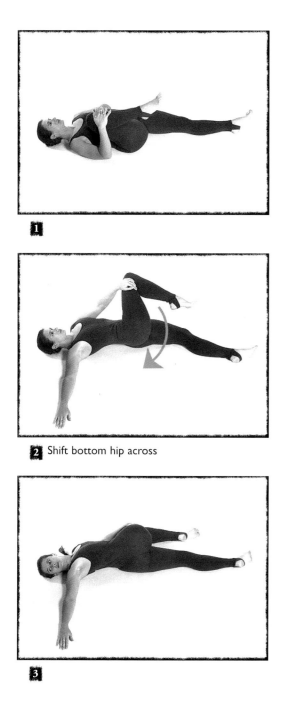

1

2 Shift bottom hip across

3

this refinement, and as a result the spine is both rotated and hyperextended (arched) in the final position, the two movements together often being sufficient to cause pain in a sore back. Generally, it is the extension component of the movement which causes the pain.

Take the top leg across slowly as far as it will go. The limit is when the opposite shoulder begins to lift off the floor. You may hold onto a sturdy table-leg to hold the shoulder down, but do not force the stretch. Concentrate on breathing and relaxing. Notice that as you breathe in the leg tends to rise and as you breathe out it tends to go closer to the floor. You may rest the knee of the bent leg on a cushion if the end position is quite a way from the floor. This will enable you to hold the position comfortably. As you become more flexible, reduce the thickness of the cushion. Look at the outstretched hand. Hold the final position for about ten breaths, and return the leg to the starting position (second photograph).

Rather than returning the leg to the floor, bring the other knee up and change your hands over to it, and then let the first leg down to the floor. Again, this will avoid hyperextending the lower back, and make the exercise more comfortable. Repeat all directions for the second leg, taking care to note the tighter side. Next time you stretch, begin with (and repeat the movement for) the tighter side.

When you are comfortable with the stretch a C–R version may be tried. In the final stretch position, hold the top leg and very gently try to press it upwards against the resistance of your hand for a few seconds. Rather than the hip muscles, use the back and waist muscles to press back in order to maximise the stretch in these muscles. Relax, breathe in, and on a breath out, slowly press the leg closer to the floor.

4. *Partner-assisted rotation*

At this point I should like to introduce the first partner exercise, which is an assisted version of the exercise you have just done. Do not attempt this partner version before doing the exercise unassisted. Unless you have done the standard version, you will not have a clear idea of your limits, and neither will your partner. If the partner has been watching your effort this far, he or she will be in a good position to assist.

Look at the photograph. You are lying on the floor, in the second position of the exercise. Your partner is kneeling (on one knee) on the side you are rotating away from. Your partner's other leg is brought up for stability (second photograph on page 177 shows this position from the other side). One hand is holding the shoulder onto the floor, and the other is placed on the top hip, ready to apply a small horizontal force. The partner must be in a stable position, and well balanced. Note the position of the hand on the shoulder: you may have to ask the partner to move the hand more onto the shoulder, or further down the arm until a comfortable position is found. One of the biceps' tendons runs across the front of the shoulder and it may be uncomfortable if much weight is put on it. Notice also that the partner has his or her weight more or less directly above the hand holding the shoulder. You move yourself into the beginning of the stretch position—not the maximum position. Ask your partner to hold you there; that is, the partner's hand placed on the hip does not push the hip further away—it merely rests there as a solid barrier. When your partner is ready, you very gently push the top hip back in the opposite direction (back against your partner's hand) while counting to ten. This is the isometric contraction discussed previously. Very little effort needs to be used here; it is more of a lean than a push in the early stages. Always be guided by your perception of pain—if it hurts you, stop pushing.

Assuming that the pushing part has been completed without a problem, stop pushing. The partner's hand at this stage has remained an immovable barrier against which you have been pushing. The next stage is the taking of a deep breath, after which you relax completely. The partner, watching and listening to your breathing, leans a small weight horizontally and slowly in the direction indicated, to take the hip a little further away. The partner must be very careful at this point, watching your face for any signs of discomfort, stopping if necessary. When a stronger but still comfortable stretch position is reached, the partner holds you there. You remain in the position for the ten-breath count, concentrating on letting any tension go. Imagine the tension is leaving the body with each breath out.

The partner must hold the final position without moving at all. The support provided by the partner must be stable and still, best provided by arranging his or her body so that the effort required can be provided by a leaning force rather than a pushing force. If you feel at all uncertain of the support, you will not permit yourself to relax. It is mainly for this reason that all partner exercises have precise directions to your partner, as well as to you.

Repeat all directions for the other side.

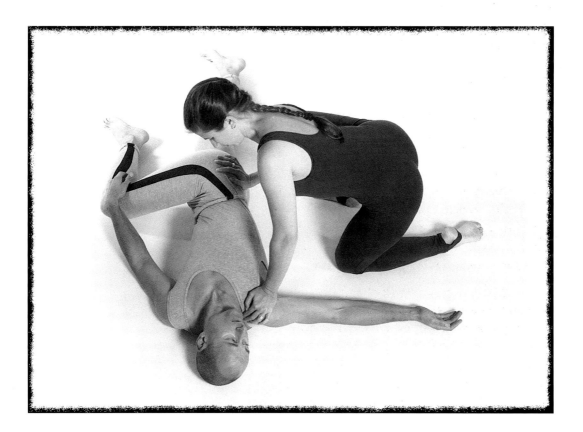

5. Rotation using chair

A similar, but more gentle, rotation can be done using the chair. Look at the photographs. Sit across the seat to prevent the hips moving (bracing the side of the leg against the chair's back). Hold the chair back with an appropriate grip. Lift your chest up until your back feels straight (doing the exercise in front of a mirror is an excellent way to check form). Use only your arms to turn your shoulders to one side until the desired stretch is felt. Repeat for the other side.

If you are careful, a C–R version can be done too. Holding yourself in a gentle stretch position, apply a light twisting force in the opposite direction using the muscles of the waist against the resistance of the arms. Stop and take in a deep breath. Relax completely and, using your arms, rotate the shoulders a little further with respect to the hips. You must keep the back straight, and you must not force this technique. You may feel the major effects of this movement a little higher in the back than with the last exercise.

If for some reason you cannot apply the necessary effort yourself, your partner may assist. The partner supports you in a moderate stretch position. Notice that the partner's arms are straight. Most people are stronger and more stable this way, using the muscles of the waist and hips in preference to the muscles of the arms. The partner's hand and arm positions are shown in the photographs. Essentially the same technique is used in the partner C–R version. You twist gently back against the restraint provided by the partner, who does not permit your shoulders to move. Do this for ten seconds or so. You then stop pushing and take in a deep breath. As you breathe out, your partner takes the shoulders a little further in the stretch direction. The partner holds you in the final position for five breaths or so, or about thirty seconds. Repeat for the other side. This is an excellent middle back stretch.

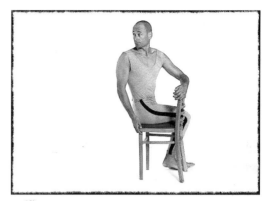

1

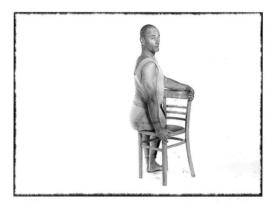

2

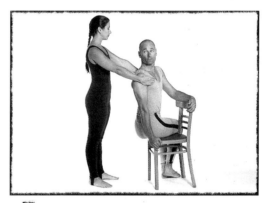

3

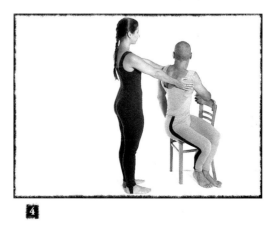

4

6. *Hands and knees* (cat) *pose*

This minor pose is often used to relax the lower and middle back muscles after backward bending, but is included because it is a gentle and safe stretch in its own right. It is sometimes called the *cat* pose, because the shapes resemble the sort of stretches cats do upon awakening. I have added a strengthening component, and a lateral flexion (bend to the side) to the normal spinal flexion movement.

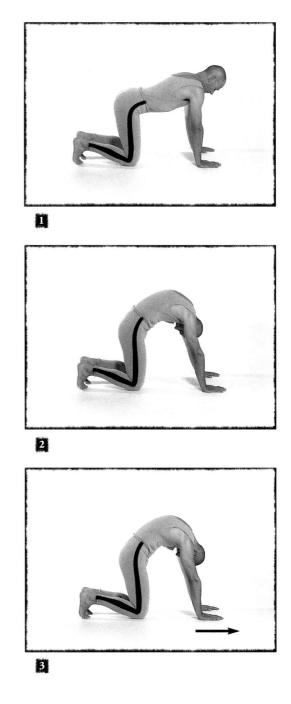

Begin by kneeling on the floor. If the knees feel uncomfortable, kneel on a folded towel or the like—you cannot stretch properly if you are being distracted by discomfort anywhere in the body. Notice that the knees are under the hips, and the hands are slightly in front of the shoulders. Let the head slowly hang down under its own weight. When it has descended as far as it can, draw the chin into the chest. Feeling your weight evenly on hands and knees, slowly curl the body as shown. This requires the stomach (abdominal) muscles to be contracted. Take your time doing this, both to feel the stretch and to be aware of the location of the muscles being used.

If you wish to make the stretch stronger, use the muscles of the shoulders to push the hands away from you, gently, as though you were trying to slide them away while contracting the stomach muscles. This extra effort increases the stretch in the middle and, for some people, the upper back. Hold for ten breaths in and out. Note that breathing will be difficult because the abdominal area is contracted and lung volume reduced. Return to the starting position.

In the relaxed hands-and-knees position, slowly look around behind you, trying to see the heel of the foot on the side to which you are turning. Feel the contraction of the waist muscles on this side. This movement stretches the same muscle groups on the opposite side of the body. See if you can feel this. Repeat for the other side, and after holding the final position for a few seconds, briefly return to the first stretch position, and back to the starting position. The reason for returning briefly to the first stretch position is to relax the muscles which need to contract to produce the stretch position.

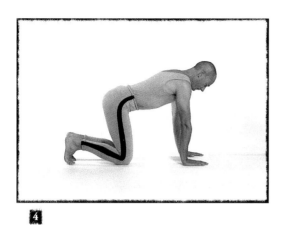

4

The advice to stretch a second time on the side you begin with is a general rule for the whole body. When stretching matched pairs of muscles which require the contraction of one of the pairs to produce the stretch in the other, you will benefit from repeating the first side's stretch briefly, to relax the last-used muscle group.

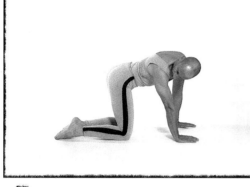

5

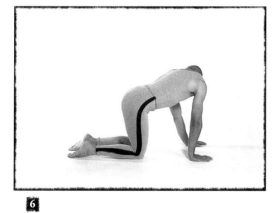

6

7. *Iliopsoas (modified* salute to the sun)

This stretch is very effective for relieving low-back pain, even though it does not stretch the lower back in any way. It stretches a group of powerful muscles, the hip flexors (particularly *psoas major* and *iliacus*), shown in the illustrations overleaf. These muscles can play a major role in shaping the lumbar curve, especially if the abdominal muscles are weak. Inflexible hip flexors are often the reason people with back problems cannot lie face up with legs outstretched without feeling discomfort. These muscle groups are also often implicated in athletes with low-back pain, especially those who use incorrect strengthening exercises for the abdominal muscles (see chapter three).

Anatomically, the action of the hip flexors is to pull the knee to the chest (ignoring the abdominal muscles for a moment). Accordingly, to stretch the flexors the thigh needs to be taken backwards with respect to the trunk. Look at the photograph of the starting position: I am kneeling on one leg, which has been placed as far back as it will go (we will refer to this as the *back* leg), and supporting the remainder of the body's weight on the other leg (the *front* leg). Notice that the foot of the front leg is well in front of the knee. Place the hand on the bottom, directly behind the hip joint and with the elbow pointing backwards, as shown. Use this hand to push the hip of the back leg forwards as far as it will go—this requires that this hip rotates away from, and in front of, the pushing hand. This direction is crucial: if the hips are not in the recommended position, the thigh muscles, rather than the hip flexors, will be stretched. To be specific, the starting position requires that the hip joints be square (at 90 degrees) to the line of the legs or, if sufficiently flexible, the back leg's hip slightly ahead of the other hip, as seen from above.

With the back leg's hip rotated forwards (and held in this position for the duration of the exercise), keep the body vertical by placing your other hand on the knee of the front leg, as shown. If balance is difficult, support yourself by placing this hand on a chair, or a wall. Let both hips sink in the direction of the floor, only as far as you can maintain both the forward rotation of the back hip and the trunk's alignment with respect to the floor. Neither of these constraints may be sacrificed to achieve a lower position.

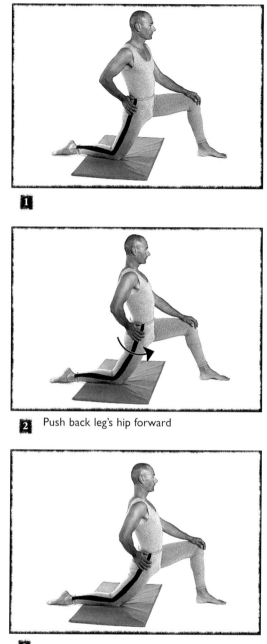

1

2 Push back leg's hip forward

3

Sinking towards the floor takes the back leg away behind the body, with the main stretch being felt at the front of the back leg, high up near the hip joint. You may also feel a stretch at the back of the front leg. Remain in the stretch position for the usual ten breath period, and use the arm on the front leg to help you return to the starting position. Repeat directions for the other leg. Take special notice of whether one set of hip flexors is tighter than the other. If this is the case, the next time you stretch begin with the tighter hip, and stretch it a second time after stretching the other.

If balancing in the exercise is a problem even if the width between the front foot and the back knee is adequate, you may try doing the pose with the front leg side of the body next to a wall. By leaning slightly against the wall, balancing is made easier.

Psoas, iliacus (iliopsoas), and quadratus lumborum

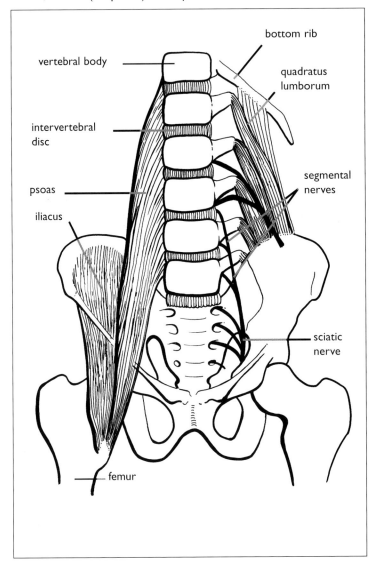

vertebral body

bottom rib

quadratus
lumborum

intervertebral
disc

segmental
nerves

psoas

iliacus

sciatic
nerve

femur

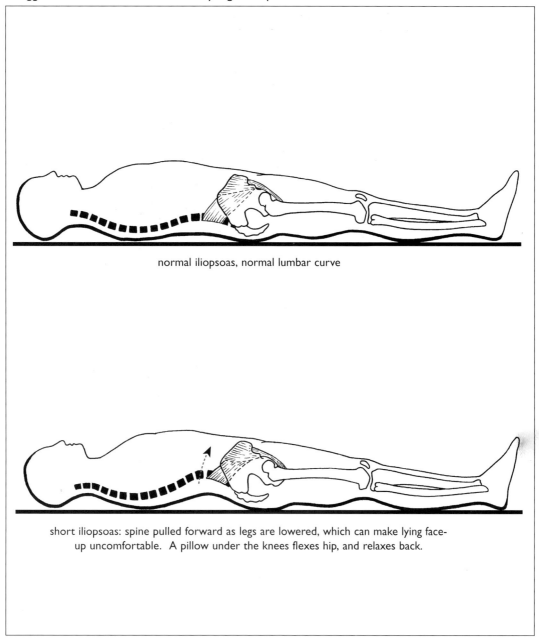

normal iliopsoas, normal lumbar curve

short iliopsoas: spine pulled forward as legs are lowered, which can make lying face-
up uncomfortable. A pillow under the knees flexes hip, and relaxes back.

8. *Middle and upper back* (rabbit) *pose*

This stretch is included in the back section, because it stretches the middle to upper back, depending on your proportions. *Trapezius* and the *rhomboids* are stretched, and the movement is also one of the few solo stretches available for a pair of muscles that lift the shoulders (*levator scapulae;* these muscle groups are shown overleaf). One end of *levator scapulae* attaches to the shoulder blade, and the other to the side of the cervical spine. Because these muscles either elevate one or both shoulders or flex the neck to one side, this exercise can also be used as an indirect neck stretching exercise.

Head placement is critical, both to avoid possible neck injury and to ensure that the stretch is felt in the correct place. Those who are very stiff may find it difficult to get into the starting position. If you cannot get into position without distorting the shape of the exercise, do not attempt it. After sufficient time practising other exercises (11 and 15, for example) you may re-attempt the movement.

Kneel down as shown. While supporting yourself with one arm, reach through the knees (notice that the knees are further apart than the ankles) and hold the foot of the same side with the indicated grip. Curl forwards and place the top of the head on the floor, and rest some of the body's weight on the head. This locates the shoulders with respect to the hips. Now reach through the knees with the other hand, and hold the other foot. Ensure that the top of the head is resting on the floor. Breathe normally. Gripping the feet firmly, slowly and gently push the hips forward. Because the hands are holding the feet, the middle and upper back are drawn into a forward stretch, as in drawing a bow. Generally, this will not irritate the lower back if back pain is your problem—all of the stretch is higher in the back.

In the final position, breathe in and out for five breaths or so. Let the stretch go by letting the hips return to the start position. Take one hand off one foot, and place it in the support position. Now breathe in, and hold your breath while you use the support hand to lift yourself back to the beginning position. When there, resume normal breathing. Do not lift yourself up into the start position using the muscles of the back. As a general rule,

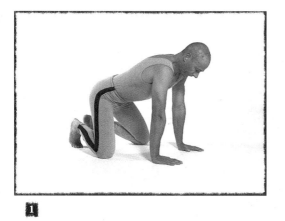

1

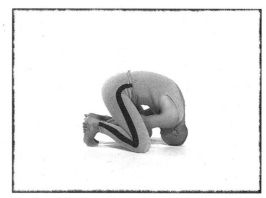

5

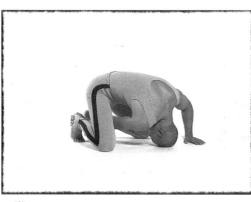

2

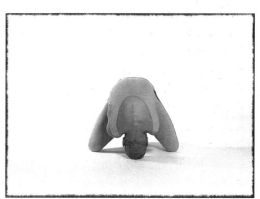

6

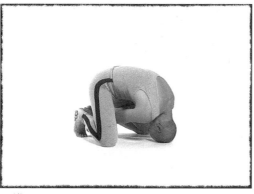

3

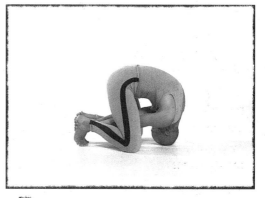

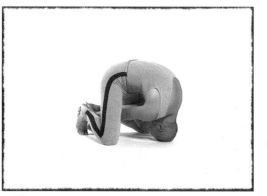

4

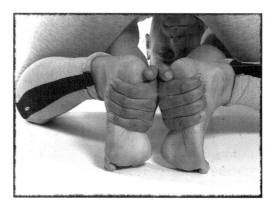

when returning from any extended (stretched) position, use muscles other than the ones you have been stretching.

Two C–R stretches may be done. When in the stretch position (either version) try to shrug the shoulders while holding firmly onto the feet. This engages *levator scapulae* and consequently a stronger stretch will be felt in these muscles. In the second C–R stretch, try to draw the shoulder blades together directly behind you while holding the feet firmly. Restretching will concentrate the effects in *trapezius* and the *rhomboids*.

You may move the main locus of the stretch further down to the middle of the back by holding the feet from outside the legs. Here you will need to have the knees a little closer together than the feet so that you can hold the feet without interference. All other directions are the same.

Levator scapulae spans cervical vertebrae and shoulder blade

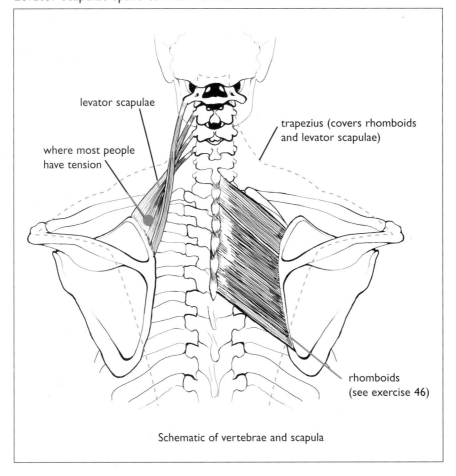

levator scapulae

trapezius (covers rhomboids and levator scapulae)

where most people have tension

rhomboids
(see exercise 46)

Schematic of vertebrae and scapula

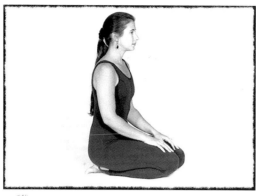

 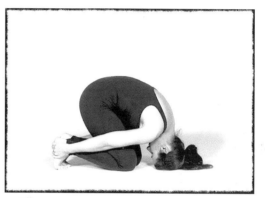

 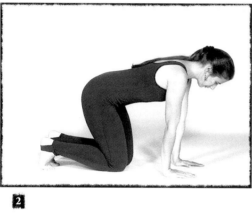

 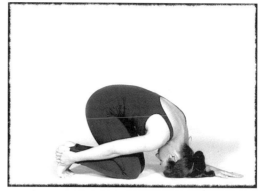

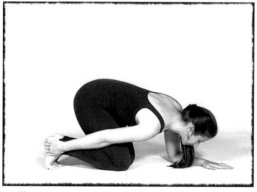

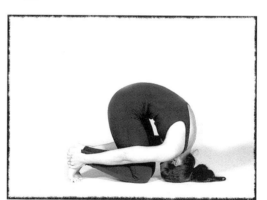

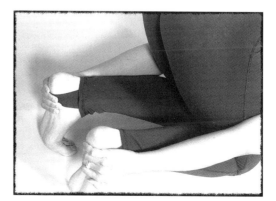

9. Hip

Inflexible hip muscles (in particular *gluteus maximus*, the main muscles of the bottom, and *piriformis*, one of the external hip rotators) can contribute significantly to back pain in some people. The significance of *piriformis* with respect to back pain and sciatica is further discussed in exercise 36. This stretch is one of the best to loosen this area. It is offered in two forms.

The easier of the two, and the one which you should use if you are not sure how loose the hip joint is in this movement, begins by sitting on the floor as shown. Ensure that your weight is placed evenly on both bottom bones (the *ischial tuberosities*), with one leg extended. Bend the other leg at the knee and place the foot on the outside of the outstretched leg. If sciatica or hamstring tightness prevents you from sitting upright with one leg extended, place a cushion or similar under the knee of the straight leg or sit on a table with the extended leg hanging over the edge as shown (bottom photograph, left column). Flexing the knee in these ways relieves the stretch on the hamstrings. Check that your back is held straight (lift the chest to make sure), and grasp the knee with the crook of the elbow of the shoulder opposite the bent knee. As you breathe out, gently bring the knee back to the chest. You will feel the stretch in the hip of the held leg. Stretch the other side.

If one hip is tighter in this movement (likely to be the case if you have a leg-length difference) a contraction may be used on the tight hip to minimise the difference in function. Gently press the leg away from the body while holding it in the stretched position for a few seconds, and relax completely. Check the back for straightness, and while breathing out, gently restretch the hip by bringing the knee towards the body. Hold the final position for five breaths or so. Do not press the knee away from the body with any great force—a gentle press will do the same job with less discomfort.

In all respects other than the starting position, the second version is the same as the first. Look at the photograph. Do not sit on the folded lower leg, but keep it sufficiently outside the line of the body to permit both bottom bones to contact the floor firmly. Because this is an important point, you may wish to try this version sitting on a hard floor without any mat or cushion the first few times you try the exercise. Move subtly from side to side in the starting position until you are sure that both bones are pressing on the floor equally. Follow the directions for the above exercise, including those for the C–R component.

This completes our rehabilitation back exercises.

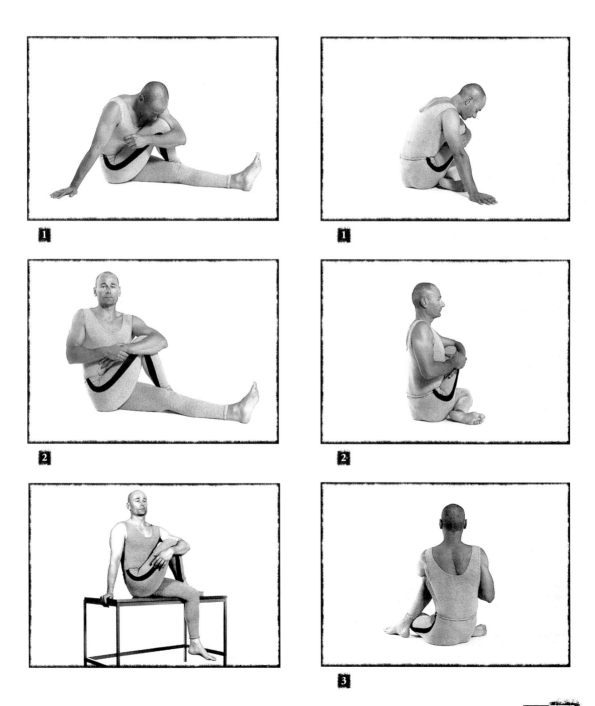

NECK STRETCHING EXERCISES (REHABILITATION AND PREVENTION)

10. *Partner shoulder depress (chair)*

Caution: those who suffer from any sort of lower back problem which renders them unduly sensitive to axial (longitudinal) compression of the spine should approach this exercise with great care.

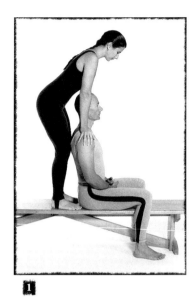

Of all the stretches presented in my exercise classes, this is the most popular. It makes everyone feel lighter, as though their cares have been lifted from their shoulders. In fact, as this movement stretches the muscles which hold the shoulders in their usual position, this is both literally and metaphorically true. This exercise is a particular boon for people who spend much of their life at a keyboard or hunched over books.

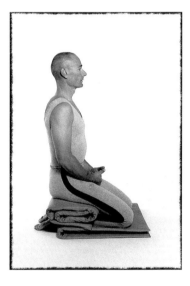

As we become more tense, or as we are exposed to any frustrating experience, the shoulders move upward of their own accord. The muscles between the shoulders and neck become tight and painful. This reaction is apparently universal, and over time, may lead to conditions such as 'frozen shoulders'. Tension in these muscles is nearly always present in patients with neck pain, and the same tension invariably accompanies conditions such as Repetitive Strain Injury (now known as Occupational Overuse Syndrome). Tension in the *levator scapulae* and *scalene* muscles always seems to be an accompanying phenomenon, the successful reduction of which alleviates much of the neck pain as well. Recall the last really relaxed person you saw: there would have been much open space between the ears and the shoulders, suggesting that (other things being equal) relaxed people carry their shoulders lower than those who are not. Angry people hold their shoulders up around their ears. This exercise will remove tension from this area. See exercise 13 for further stretches for *levator scapulae* and the *scalene* muscles.

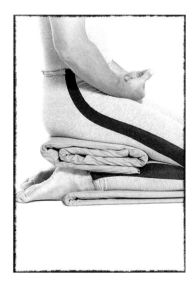

Look at the photograph. We are using a bench for ease of illustration, but you can use two strong (but non-sliding) chairs. This time you are sitting more conventionally, further back towards the chair back. Sit with your back straight and your shoulders relaxed into their lowest position. Your partner stands on a similarly strong chair (one which can support their whole weight), bends his or her knees slightly, inclines forward from the hips, and places straight arms (hands and fingers lightly cupping your shoulders) as shown. Once comfortable and secure in this

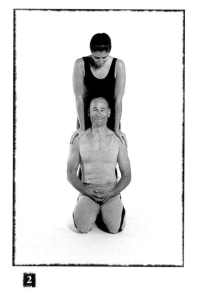

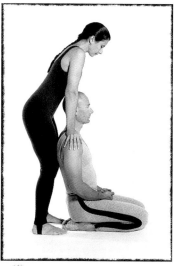

position, the partner leans forward from the waist so that some of his or her weight is transferred evenly to both your shoulders. Doing the exercise in front of a mirror to check the level of the shoulders is helpful.

Your partner must not push your shoulders down with his or her strength, but should lean some weight on you, enough so that you feel a stretch in the muscles mentioned. Your partner's weight must only push your shoulders towards the floor, not bend your back forwards. Accordingly, you need to hold your upper body straight while letting the shoulders be stretched. Once you have let yourself relax in the stretch position, ask your partner to hold the shoulders there; that is, to resist your attempts to lift the shoulders. When your partner is ready, slowly lift your shoulders moderately strongly (the partner resisting all the while) for ten seconds or so. Your partner must not allow the shoulders to move. When you have completed the contraction phase, warn your partner that you are about to stop lifting, and do so. (The warning is so that your partner removes some of the weight from your shoulders when you stop, so that they do not end up on top of you).

Take a deep breath and, letting the shoulders relax completely, ask the partner to lean on you once more. You will find that the shoulders drop quite dramatically, giving you a pleasing stretch in an area which most people find extremely difficult to stretch. Repeat the lifting–holding–relaxing sequence, up to a total of three times—beyond this, any additional effect is usually negligible. To finish, the partner removes their weight, and you lift the shoulders up and down, letting them drop down.

Notice from the photographs that the exercise may be done from the kneeling seated position if this is comfortable for you. No strain should be felt in the knees in this position. A firm pillow or similar object placed between the bottom and the heels will help the legs feel comfortable. If there is too much stretch in the insteps (from being stretched backward), sit across a cushion in such as way as to relieve the instep and toes; a second cushion goes between the bottom and the heels as before.

In the kneeling version, you should lean backwards against your partner's knees for support, but do not exaggerate this. All other directions are the same as the chair version.

11. Chin to chest, using chair, C–R

The purpose of this exercise is to stretch the muscles controlling extension of the neck; that is, to stretch the muscles that are supporting the head as you read this book (assuming that you are reading in the conventional, upright seated position). The anatomy of the neck is complex, but for the present purpose it is enough to draw your attention to a few basic points. When we incline the head forward, the neck may bend anywhere along its length. What we want is for the load of the head (which is quite considerable) to be distributed along the whole of the neck—not merely in one or two places. Thus we shall need to monitor the shape the neck makes as we bend it. A dressing mirror is ideal, set at an angle that permits the side of the neck to be seen (placing it to your front at about 45 degrees to the side is effective). Specifically, what we want to avoid is an inclination of the head that is achieved only by tilting it forward on the neck. Bending in this fashion involves only the top two vertebrae, and will not stretch all the back neck muscles.

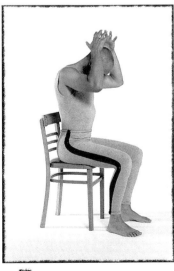

The best way to achieve the desired stretch is both to watch the shape of the neck and to feel where the stretch is being experienced along it. However, it is possible to feel the stretch in only one small local area along the back of the neck even though the curve in the neck seems to be ideal. This may only mean that this is the place where you hold the most tension.

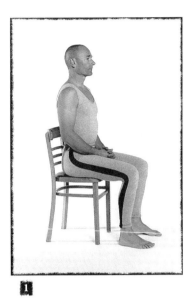

Incline the head forward, trying to divide the movement into tilting of the head and bending the neck itself. When you have reached a position of stretch, hold it for a few breaths in and out, letting the tension go. When you have relaxed sufficiently, place your clasped hands on what is now the top of your head (somewhere behind where the top normally is) and gently let the weight of the arms rest on the head. Let this weight come onto the back of the neck slowly, so that if the stretch becomes too strong you can remove the arms' weight before you hurt yourself. As the weight is felt, the head will incline further towards the chest. Feel the stretch, visualising the tension leaving the body with each breath out, and try to feel the stretch over as much of the back of the neck as possible. ('Visualising' means trying to see clearly in your mind that the tension you feel is moving out of the place you feel it, and is leaving the body with each breath out. Visualisation is discussed in more detail in chapter five.) Stay in the final position for five to ten breaths.

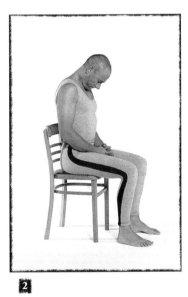

To come out of the stretch, remove the hands from the top of the head, slowly lift the head to the neutral position, and rest.

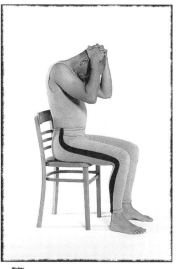

4

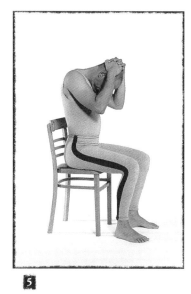
5

There are two C–R stretches, both requiring care. Once the neck muscles are accustomed to the weight of the arms on the back of the neck, very gently push the head back against the resistance of your hands for a few seconds. Remove the hands for a second or two, then replace them. While breathing out, restretch extremely cautiously. Hold the final position for five breaths.

In the second C–R stretch, very gently try to tilt the head backwards, by trying to lift the chin in the stretch position rather than pushing the whole head backwards. On a breath out, restretch carefully. This latter version activates the small muscles under the back of the skull (the *suboccipitals*). Holding tension in these muscles can lead to the familiar 'tension headaches.'

After stretching forwards, it is good to stretch backwards briefly and gently, and to restretch forwards for a moment. This makes the neck feel most comfortable (in contrast with only stretching forwards). The safest way, after you have come back to the starting position, is to open the mouth wide, keep the shoulders relaxed, and slowly tilt the head backwards as far as you can. When in the final stretch position, gently close the teeth together. Keep the back straight—do not confuse leaning backwards with stretching the neck. Closing the teeth after you have moved the head backwards helps concentrate the stretch in the muscles and skin at the front of the throat, and reduces any uncomfortable compression in the joints of the spine at the back of the neck.

Once in the final stretch position, you may incline the head gently to one side. So doing will stretch the front neck muscles on the side of the neck you are stretching away from. Hold the new position for a breath or two, slowly incline the head to the other side, and hold for the same duration. Check to see if there are any left-right differences.

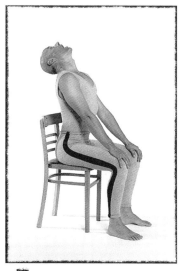
6

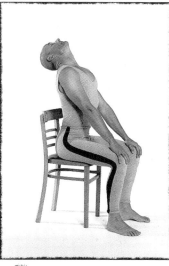
7 Incline left and right from this position

12. Neck extension over support

If inclining the head backwards is painful for you, there is a technique that takes some of the compression load off sensitive joints. It also allows you to control the extent of backwards movement completely, using your hands.

Look at the photographs. Here I am using the end of the bench with a few mats for padding to simulate a firm mattress as a shelf over which to hang my head. If your neck is extremely sensitive to being moved backwards, do not have your shoulders as far towards the edge. Use the tendency for the edge of the mattress to give way under your weight as a gentle support for most of the length of the neck.

While holding your head, completely supported by your hands, approach the edge of the mattress. At this stage, the neck and head should be in the anatomically neutral position, although horizontal. Settle yourself, take a breath in and, very gently and slowly, lower the head (with respect to the surface of the mattress) a small distance. In this version of backwards neck bending, do not have the mouth open. The purpose here is to lower the neck back only until these muscles are stretched. Doing the exercise with the mouth closed will reduce the backward movement of the head and neck somewhat. The important point is to control the movement using your hands. When in the final position, count five breaths, and return the head to the normal position using the hands, then hold the head until you move away from the edge of the mattress.

Once familiar with the movement, you may add a rotation component if you are careful. In the final stretch position, gently turn the head a small amount to one side, and hold that position. Experiment to find the amount of turn that gives you the best stretch on the front and side of the neck. Repeat for the other side. Once you have completed the exercise and you are sitting up, briefly stretch forwards for a few seconds to make the neck feel comfortable.

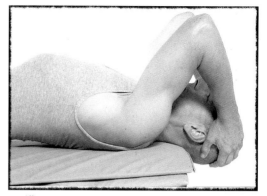

2

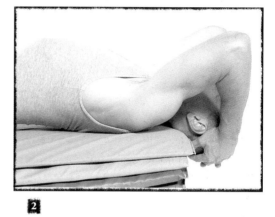

1

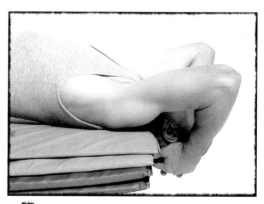

3

13. Lateral neck flexion, using chair, C–R

Much neck pain is felt in the side of the neck, and most often on the dominant side, indicated by left or right handedness. This exercise will stretch some of the muscles involved, and is a complement to the first exercise of this section (the one where your partner leans down on your shoulders). The last version of this exercise can be used to stretch the three *scalene* muscles. Excessive tension in these muscles can cause thoracic outlet compression syndrome, giving rise to referred pain in the front or back of the arm, upper medial border of the shoulder blade, and numbness in the fingers. Two C–R stretches are offered in each version.

As you will know (and certainly will see if you watch yourself), bending the neck to the side is usually achieved in part by lifting the shoulder we are stretching away from and by inclining the whole body. Knowing this, we can concentrate the stretch in the side neck muscles by restraining the shoulder we are stretching away from.

The aim is to stretch away from one shoulder. Hold the seat of the chair with the hand of that shoulder. Keep the back straight (as seen from the side). If you have a tendency to be a little hunched over, breathe in and lift the chest before you begin and hold the body straight during the exercise. Watch yourself—as you lift the chest, the upper back straightens. Ensure that the head is over the shoulders, as it might be seen from the side.

Now, incline the head to the side, away from the restrained shoulder. Here too we are trying to make the whole neck curve to the side, and for this reason I am holding a credit card between the teeth to illustrate the inclination of the head on the neck and the curve of the neck to the side. Avoid doing only one or the other. Do not rotate the head or incline the neck forwards. The movement ideally occurs in one plane only, the vertical plane going through both shoulders. The stretch will be felt in the side of the neck, anywhere from the shoulder to the ear.

The next part requires care. When in the fully-stretched position, and after having held this position for three or four breaths in and out, reach up with the free hand and place two fingers on the side of the head above the ear as shown. Very gently press these fingers onto the side of the head to increase the stretch fractionally. Hold the final position for a few breaths. This must be done extremely sensitively. Err on the side of not using enough pressure.

Alternatively, you can use contractions to enhance the stretch effects, if you are careful. Rather than using the fingers to stretch

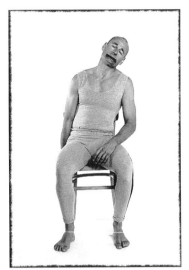

1 Version 1 (sideways only)

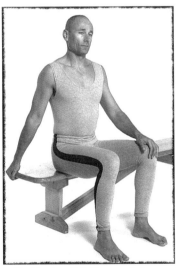

1 Version 2 (sideways & forwards)

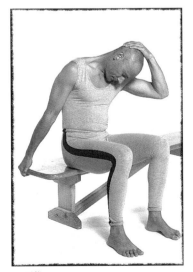

4

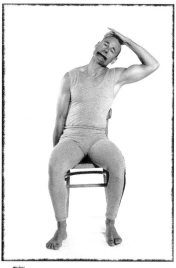

2

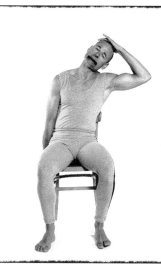

3

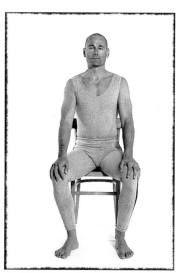

4

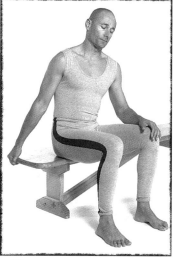

2

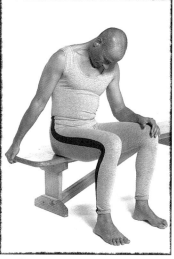

3

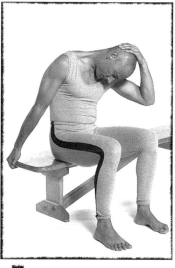

5

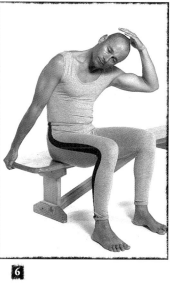

6

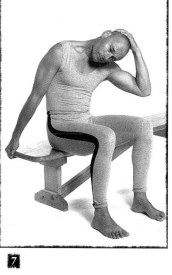

7

the neck further, place the two fingers on the head as instructed, but this time use the fingers only to locate the head. In the first contraction, try to shrug the shoulder of the restraining hand for a few seconds. Stop shrugging, take a breath in, and on a breath out lean the body further away from the restraining hand. This will stretch you above the shoulder. For the second C–R, gently press the head back against your fingers for a few seconds. Stop pressing, and take the fingers from the head for a second or two. Replace the fingers, and while breathing out, very gently restretch. Hold the final position for five breaths in and out. Repeat for the other side. These C–R stretches may be used singly or together.

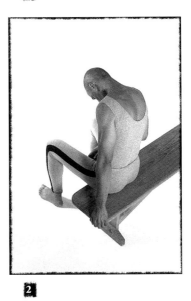

A second version of this exercise is offered, and is a particularly effective stretch. It is a combination of forward and sidewards bending (flexion and lateral flexion) with a small rotation, depending on where you wish to feel the stretch. The directions are complicated, but no other neck stretch will leave the neck feeling as good as this one will. Examine the photographs carefully before trying it for the first time, and note the directions of the assistance movements.

Begin as before, restraining the shoulder by holding onto the seat of the chair, but with the hand a little further back than before. Experiment with placement—ten centimetres behind the hip joint is a good starting position. Lean both to the side and slightly forwards. This will mean directly away from the hand restraining the shoulder. Let the head go forwards onto the chest, then take the head to the side. At this point, the head will be directly opposite the restraining hand, meaning that the neck is both flexed and laterally flexed.

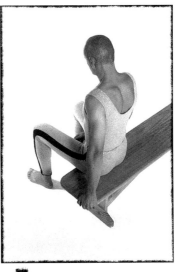

Now reach up with the other hand, and place two fingers on the head, opposite the restraining hand. To focus the stretch exactly where you need it, try turning the head slightly to the side of the restraining hand. Once the spot is located, use both C–R stretches, the first by shrugging the shoulder of the hand holding the support, and the second by gently pressing back against the fingers using the muscles you feel the stretch in. To finish, restretch using the fingers on the head, and hold the final position for five breaths. Repeat for the other side.

To stretch the *scalenes* a similar approach is used (not shown). Hold the support about ten centimetres *in front of* the hip joint, and lean the head *back and to the side*, away from the hand. Both C–R stretches are used as before. Slightly turning the head away from, or towards, the restraining hand will locate the most effective stretch positions.

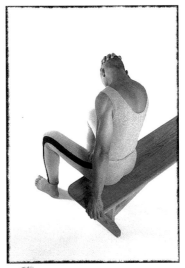

3 Version 2, from behind

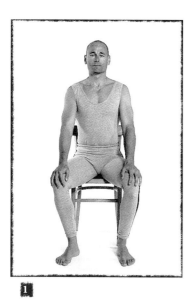

1

2

14. Neck rotation

This stretch demonstrates how much your normal pattern of movement constrains your flexibility. Look at the photograph. Sit squarely on the chair, with your weight evenly on both bottom bones, leaning neither forwards nor backwards, with your back straight and body relaxed. Slowly turn your head to one side without inclining it forwards and without tilting it to the side. The movement is pure rotation. Turn the head as far as you can, and when it will go no further, hold the final position. Pause, take a deep breath in, and as you exhale, try to turn the head further. Considerable extra movement will be achieved with the second effort. Hold the final position for a few breaths in and out, and feel the muscles being stretched (at the side of the neck you are stretching away from) and the muscles you are using (at the side of the neck and between the neck and the shoulder you are stretching towards). Repeat for the other side, but finish with a brief rotation towards the side you stretched first, to release the muscles you used to achieve the second movement.

The interesting aspect of this exercise is that even if you know that you will be able to turn further with a second effort, the head will not go beyond a certain position when you turn it the first time. A second effort usually produces further movement, however. This suggests that flexibility is a phenomenon deriving both from structure and patterns of use; in other words, a neuromuscular phenomenon. With respect to any left-right difference found in this exercise, a question to ask may be over which shoulder do you look as you back your car out of the garage each day?

15. *Chin-on-chest variations; chair (two movements)*

These two movements complete the rehabilitation neck movements. They are to be done only if the preceding neck exercises can be done without discomfort.

Both exercises begin with the same starting position. Sit up straight, towards the front of the chair, with your feet underneath your knees for stability. Let the chin move forward towards the centre of the chest, or as far as it will go. Clasp your hands together and place them on what is now the top of the head. Allow the weight of the completely relaxed arms to rest on the head. Notice that the elbows hang down; they are not held out to the sides—if they are, you are not permitting the full weight of the arms to do its job.

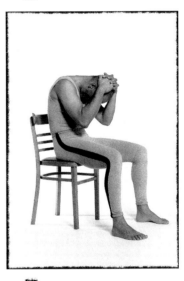

The movements are somewhat complicated, as we will be moving in a number of planes at once. Take a moment to consider the photographs—it helps a great deal to be able to visualise a movement before it is performed.

In the first movement, having assumed the starting position and moved into the stretched position, you slowly rotate at the waist. Rotate until your elbows are above either side of one knee, or until you feel a stretch down the side of the neck you are stretching away from. This should be felt all the way to the top of the shoulder blade. Hold this second position for a few breaths. This movement is a strong stretch for *levator scapulae* in particular.

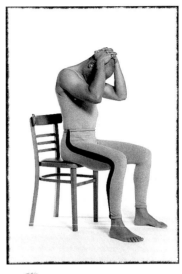

The second movement achieves an additional stretch by letting the hips roll backwards while holding the previous stretch. This curving of the spine allows you to stretch further down the back, and increases the stretch in the previously-mentioned muscles. Hold the final position for a few breaths.

Remove the hands from the head, and only then return to the starting position. The reason for this direction is that because you are stretching you are out of the normal working range of the muscles. Potentially, the neck muscles could be strained if they are used to lift both the weight of the arms and the head at the same time. Repeat for the other side of the neck.

The second exercise begins the same way, except that you may wish to have the knees a little further apart for sideways stability. After assuming the first stretch position, incline the whole upper body to one side, as close to purely sideways (that is, the plane of the shoulders) as you can. Notice that as the body inclines sidewards, the lower arm drops away from the head while the other rests on it. If this does not happen, the weight of the top

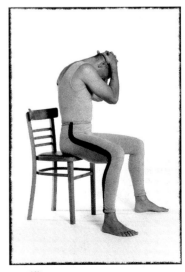

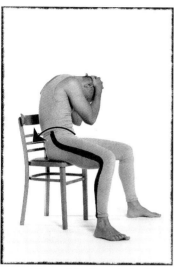

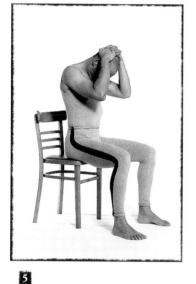

4 Hips roll backwards, body slumps forwards

5

arm will not be felt properly. The stretch will be felt in the side of the neck you are stretching away from, but closer to the ear than the previous exercise. After holding the final position for a few breaths in and out, remove the arms from the head, and only then return to the start position. Repeat for the other side.

Exercise 15 may be added to exercise 11, once you are familiar with all the components. Do the two C–R versions of exercise 11, stretch backwards and lift the shoulders up and down a couple of times to relax the muscles. Do exercise 14, and follow with the two main parts of exercise 15. C–R stretches may be added to all parts of exercise 15, wherever you find a tight muscle. I have shown the exercises in idealised forms for teaching convenience, but there are many intermediate positions between stretching forwards and sideways where you might find an excellent stretch. Exercise 13, particularly version 2, may be used at the keyboard any time for immediate relief of tension in the neck and shoulder area.

This completes the rehabilitation neck stretching exercises.

6

PLANNING A STRETCHING ROUTINE

How often, and how many times, should one do the stretches described in this and the next chapter? As a general rule, do them no less than twice a week, and no more than three times a week, but these recommendations need some qualification.

When teaching yoga and stretching in Japan, I had the opportunity to test the often-voiced claim that stretching needs to be done daily to be effective. I had groups of students working out every day, every second day, every third day, and once a week. To my surprise, the once-every-three-days group made noticeably faster progress over six months than the other groups. The next best group was the once-a-week group, and the other two groups (every day and every second day) made similar progress.

Claims regarding the necessity of daily stretching are often made, but the reasons in each case are not usually made clear, and confusion results. For example, yoga teachers recommend daily practice because one aspect of the poses is devotional. The poses are based in Indian mythology and have practical and symbolic lessons for the practitioner. Doing the poses with these ideas in mind, coupled with particular ways of breathing, helps the mind focus on these lessons. As the goal of yoga is enlightenment, daily practice is recommended. Because of this goal, in an important sense the increased flexibility of the yoga practitioner is a by-product of the practice rather than being its main focus.

In dance and gymnastics, daily practice of stretching exercise is also recommended, although for different reasons. However, these disciplines distinguish between limber classes, which loosen up the body in preparation for the day's skill classes, and stretching, which is designed to increase the range of movement. In practice, these distinctions are often blurred and the individual concerned decides which of these goals will be pursued on any given day on an ad hoc basis according to how he or she feels.

Your goals can be stated clearly. You are trying to reduce your neck or back pain, and we are assuming that the right stretching exercise will help. Once you have chosen the exercises, how often should they be done? We need to tread a fine line between doing enough to have the desired effect, but not so much that you further irritate the parts of the body concerned. Every second day is the right frequency to begin with, while being prepared to modify this as you monitor the effects of the exercise. If, for example, you do the chair exercise (the first one in this chapter) and experience some relief, repeat it after a moment or two to see if a little extra movement can be achieved (and to feel the slight improvement that one almost always feels doing an exercise a second time). Do any other exercises you have chosen (once or twice), and do no more that day. When you get up the next day, see how you feel. Do no exercise on this day, but use it to monitor the effects of the previous day's exercise. Do not be surprised to feel a little muscular soreness in the places you have stretched—this is normal. Usually, muscular soreness resulting from unaccustomed stretching is quite different to the pain of the original complaint, and a sign that useful change is occurring.

On the following day, monitor the body once more, and decide whether you want to have an additional rest day (two in all) or whether you wish to try the exercises again, cautiously.

Only you can decide, and often it will not be until you try the exercises that you will be able to decide. If muscular soreness is experienced, wait another day. Remember to err on the side of caution—in the beginning it is better to do too little rather than too much. In general, the rehabilitation neck exercises can be done more frequently than the back exercises. This is more to do with the size of the muscles involved than anything else (sore small muscles seem to be less of a problem than sore large ones). Ultimately, you must judge how often to do the exercises.

Let us say that a couple of months have elapsed, and the problem seems to have improved. Now you feel ready to tackle some of the more difficult exercises found in the next chapter. Again, it is better to do too little rather than too much. It is extremely tempting to do more, because the exercises seem to be having the effect you want, but here again you will need to restrain yourself. The exercises in chapter two are generally stronger than those in chapter one, and you will need longer recovery periods to accustom yourself to their effects in the beginning. At least one rest day (and preferably two) is recommended, although if muscular soreness persists, have an extra day or two. As before, each exercise may be done twice in any stretching session.

Finally, I wish to introduce some ideas that at first may seem to contradict the previous paragraphs. Presuming that you have been able to use the rehabilitation exercises successfully, many people find that they wish to do one or two of them more regularly than what I have suggested. Is this all right? Yes, once the original problem has settled down significantly. However, in recommending this, I wish to raise a distinction I made above (between limber and stretching workouts), but with a different slant.

Dancers and gymnasts do limber workouts to regain the flexibility of the day before. These are nothing more than extended warm-ups, as preparation for difficult strength or flexibility moves in the day's training. Similarly, the average person can use some particular exercises to set themselves up for the day's activities. Some of my students and patients use a number of the exercises on a daily basis in this way, before they go to work. If you are a morning person and feel happy with exercise done this way, I see no problem. However, most people are somewhat stiff in the mornings, and somewhat less sensitive to their body's feelings. For these people, I strongly recommend that the exercises be done in the evening. See p. 154 for recommendations for 'the daily six'.

Many students have listened to me talk about recommended frequencies of stretching, and have later said that they do some exercises every day, just because they feel good to do. I support this use wholeheartedly—but, if used in this fashion, do not try to improve in any of the exercises every day. Rather, use them to take tension away from a particular problem area and to try to prevent a problem from occurring. This is merely an elaboration of that very natural tendency to stretch the body mentioned in the book's opening paragraphs, except that now you have a focus and a method. Any of the exercises may be used at the end of a day in the same way to reduce the tension acquired by the body through daily life. Again, though, distinguish between doing an exercise gently (to reduce tension and regain yesterday's looseness) and a stretching workout where you are trying to improve the range of movement of some part of the body. The latter workout will result in some muscle soreness and will require a couple of days for recovery.

PREVENTIVE STRETCHING ROUTINE

These exercises are *not* to be used by anyone suffering neck or back pain. They are to be used after the rehabilitation exercises have been successful. These are strong movements and are potentially dangerous. You must practise these movements with caution. If any sign of your previous problems arises, stop doing the new exercises for a week or so and return to the rehabilitation exercises detailed in chapter one.

16. *Chair exercise, forwards; C–R; with partner*

The first photograph shows the final position of the forward bending chair exercise detailed in chapter one. Re-read the directions if you are not sure of precisely how to get into and out of the position.

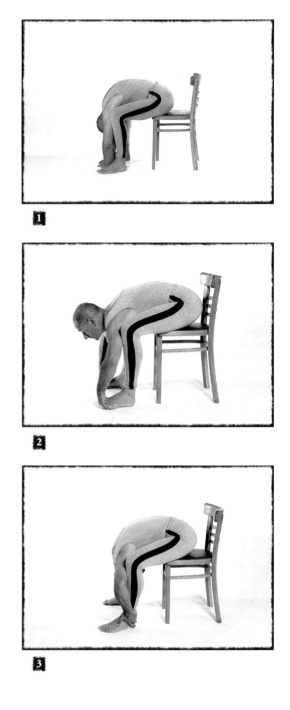

This version employs a C–R stretch for the muscles of the lumbar spine primarily, and also for the bottom, hamstring, and inner thigh muscles. Assuming that you are in a stretched position, hold onto your feet as shown (or your ankles, if you cannot reach your feet). The contraction is achieved by using the back muscles (primarily) to *try* gently to pull the hands away from the feet while not letting go of the feet, *by lifting the head and trying to arch the back backwards*. This will be an isometric contraction. To clarify: if you were to hold your back in the curved (starting) position as you try to lift the hands away from the feet, the main effect may be felt in the secondary muscles mentioned above. However, if you try to pull the hands away from the feet *by using a back straightening effort*, the main stretch effects will be felt in the muscles of the lumbar spine. To this end, before you try to pull the hands away from the feet, breathe out, lift the head away from the chest and take a *half* breathe in, and contract the back muscles against the resistance of both your arms and the combined bottom, hamstring, and inner thigh muscles, holding the contraction for a count between six and ten. This sounds more complicated than it is in practice.

This straightening effort must be small—a small, slowly and gently applied effort.

Relax the contraction, pause, breathe in deeply. As you breathe out, let the head sink forwards again and very gently use the strength of your arms to restretch the back muscles. Notice where the stretch is. You can move the

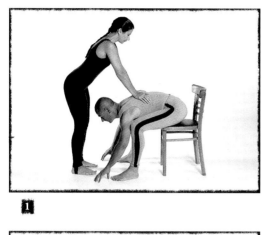

1

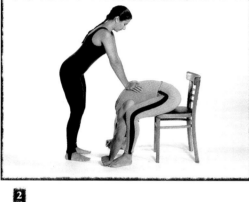

2

focus of the stretch by adjusting the force you apply (either more forwards, or more down). Remain in the final position for five breaths in and out. Come out of the position using the arms.

An even better stretch can be done with a partner, but the partner must be extremely aware and sensitive to your directions. The position of the partner's support hands is critical to feeling the stretch in the right place—the lumbar spine. Some assessment must be made by you and your partner. You will need to move into the initial stretch position, and you and your partner both look at the shape your back is making (a mirror suitably placed is effective). Aim for a smooth curve forward in the lumbar spine, from the sacrum (the lowest part of the spine) to the middle of the back. If you are tight in this area, it will appear relatively straighter than the rest of the back, or even be completely straight.

To stretch this area, your partner needs to provide support and resistance in the *middle and upper back*. This way, when you try to arch your back backwards, the effect will be concentrated in the lumbar spine. *As with the previous version, the straightening effort must be small, and applied smoothly and slowly*. Your partner takes his or her hands away from you. Stretch after the contraction by using the effort of your own arms only.

17. *Legs apart: lateral flexion with straight legs; intermediate positions*

This is one of the most important exercises in the book. It stretches most of the major muscle groups of the spine, and much else besides. It will require your best efforts and close attention to placement and alignment, but the effects are very worthwhile. I shall demonstrate it with a number of variations, but unlike some of the former movements, I shall demonstrate it in its correct (and most difficult) form *before* I discuss the easier variants, to emphasise the main principles. The exercise comprises three parts—*rotation and side bend over leg, facing leg* and *between legs*. Only the first two will be shown, because the last is an advanced move unsuitable for all but the most flexible people.

Look at the third photograph. There are a number of points to notice. Note that the shoulders are *vertical,* and *over* the leg. This position is a stretch for the muscles at the side of the waist (the *obliques*) initially, but as these muscles loosen, it becomes a powerful stretch for a muscle group commonly implicated in low back pain, *quadratus lumborum.* This muscle runs from the top of the hip bone to the sides of all the lumbar vertebrae, and a thin sheet of the muscle runs from the hip bone to the last rib. See the illustration opposite for details. As you stretch further, the muscle groups which run parallel with, and on either side of, the spine (*erector spinae,* not shown) will also be stretched.

To get into the position, sit on the floor with your legs outstretched and as far apart as you can reasonably manage. If you cannot sit as shown with a straight back (probably due to tight hamstrings or adductors) a more suitable version is described below. Lean over one leg, and hold the big toe as shown. If this is not possible, loop a towel or something similar around the foot, and hold the towel. Whichever grip you have, bend the arm and place the elbow in front of the leg you are leaning over. Press the outside of this arm against the inside of the leg, to bring the shoulder at least above, and preferably in front of, the leg. Use the elbow in this position as a brace, around which to rotate your other shoulder as far back as possible (ideally, until it is vertical, as shown). You may feel the stretch in the side

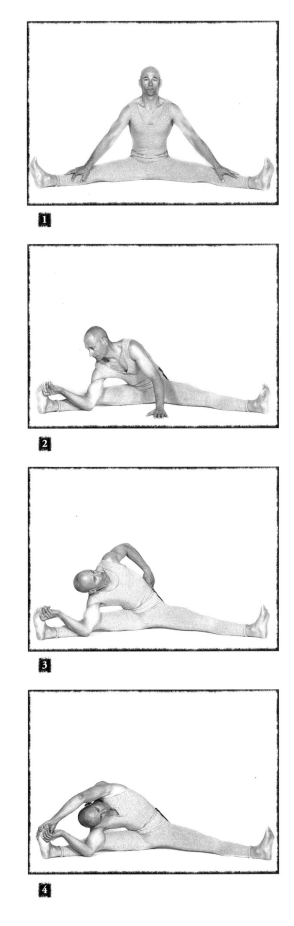

1

2

3

4

Schematic showing *quadratus lumborum,* as stretched in exercise 17

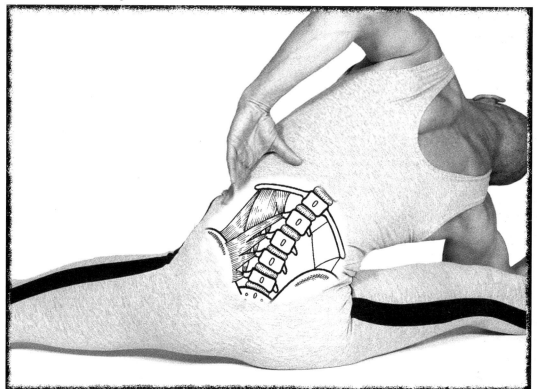

of the waist, above the hip, and along the back (and perhaps even inside) the leg you are stretching over.

When settled, and if the stretch can be increased without causing discomfort, reach out the arm of the top shoulder, in the direction of the held foot. This is the complete position. You can see that it is a rotation for the waist, a lateral flexion of the spine, and a hamstring stretch. Breathe normally in your final position for a full ten breaths or more. To come out of the stretch (and also to move the stretch closer in to the spine), very slowly roll the top shoulder forwards while maintaining the stretch as much as you can. When the stretch disappears completely, straighten up and rest for a moment. Repeat for the other leg.

Exercise 17, back and side views

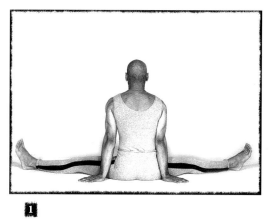
1

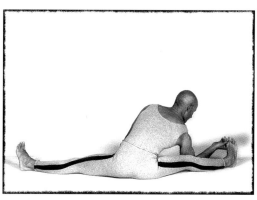
2

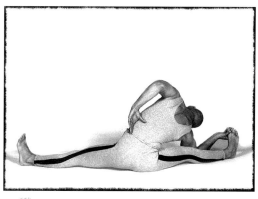
3

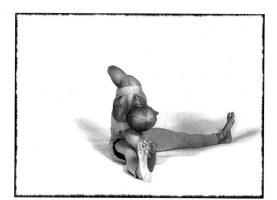
4

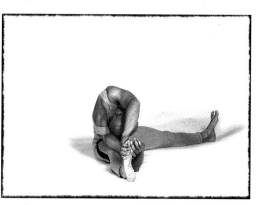
5

18. *C–R and partner version of legs* apart; *flexed knee*

The C–R version is an advanced exercise; caution is essential. Read the directions for *all* versions of the exercise before attempting one you believe to be suitable for you.

Although an advanced technique, this version is suitable for beginners *if you have a considerate partner*, and will permit the loosening of these muscles in a way which is hard to achieve on your own. The C–R version has two parts—selection of the appropriate part depends on your particular pattern of flexibility.

If you cannot put the shoulders in the suggested vertical position, have your partner support the bottom shoulder as shown. Notice that the partner's knee is supporting the bottom hand—a partner's position must always be strong and stable. Once in position, try to bring the top shoulder back. When you have reached your limit, your partner holds the top shoulder as shown while supporting the bottom one with his or her other hand. Your partner gently brings the top shoulder back until it is vertical or until the stretch is sufficient; whichever occurs first. The contraction, if desired, is that once in the final position, you ask the partner to hold you in it while you try to bring the top shoulder *forward* a little against this resistance. Hold the contraction for six to ten seconds. Relax completely, and as a separate movement (using a breath out), ask the partner to take the top shoulder back very gently until the desired stretch is felt. Repeat for the other side.

If the vertical shoulders position is not difficult, but the bend over the leg is, then use your partner's assistance in the following way. Look at the photograph (top of next page). Here, my partner has placed herself so that she can lend some weight *in the direction of the leg I am trying to bend over*. This is crucial. In this C–R version, position yourself as far in the stretch direction as you can, and when you require the assistance, ask the partner to place his or her hands on the side of your body below the top shoulder, and *in line with the leg you are trying to bend over*. Once supported, very gently push back against your partner, so that you have to use the muscles of the side of the waist and above the hip. Only push

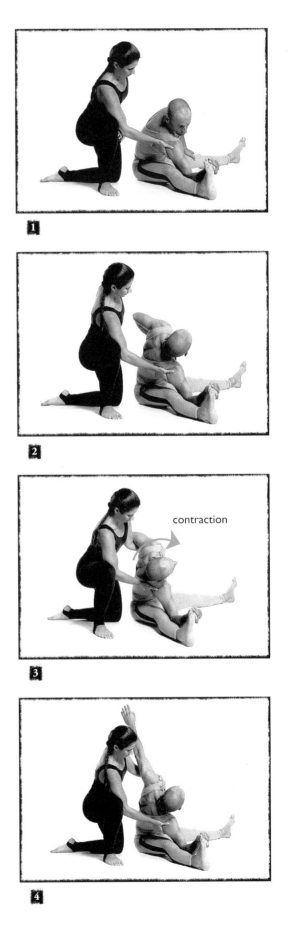

contraction

1

2

3

4

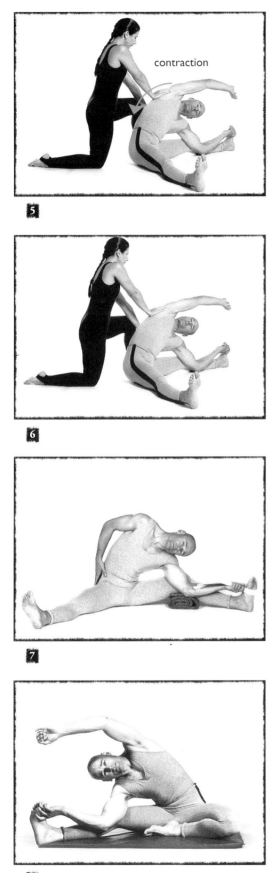

5 contraction

6

7

8

back with a small effort, which you hold for six to ten seconds. Upon relaxing, take a deep breath in, and as you breathe out, ask the partner to lean a fraction more weight on you in the direction of the leg, until you feel the right intensity of stretch. Hold the final position for the usual ten breaths. Repeat for the other side.

If the hamstring muscles are so tight that the first position is not comfortable, the movement can still be performed, albeit in a modified form. Similar benefits will be experienced, as far as the muscles of the waist and back are concerned. There are two ways of doing this. Try flexing the knee joint of the leg you are bending over. This may be achieved easily by placing a bolster or rolled-up pillow under the back of the knee (photograph 7). All other directions remain the same. The flexing of the knee reduces the stretch in the hamstring muscles, permits greater lateral flexion at the hip, and hence allows the waist muscles to be stretched by themselves. The rotation component remains.

If the adductor (inside leg) muscles are so tight that you cannot get the legs far enough apart to achieve the first position, a bent leg position is shown (photograph 8). This permits isolation of the waist muscles, but still with a hamstring stretch in the straight leg.

If both the hamstring and waist muscles are very tight, use the flexed-knee method just described, but place the leg you intend stretching over along a wall. After you have grasped the foot (by looping a towel around it) lean the body *back* against the wall. In this way, the wall becomes a support against which you can rotate the shoulders, and stretch the waist muscles. In this version also the leg you are bending away from may be folded as shown in the previous photograph. Other directions remain the same.Using the wall in this way also improves your sense of positioning the body. Repeat for the other side.

19. Legs apart: *hamstring, facing leg*

Let us assume you have completed the above stretch for both sides. Now you are in a position to do an isolation exercise for the hamstring muscles of one leg, and a back strengthening exercise at the same time. Look at the first photograph. Turn to *face* one leg. The shoulders are level with the floor. Hold one foot with the hand of the opposite shoulder's arm. Bring the other hand up to a position near the leg, so you can support yourself and keep the *centre* of your body over the leg. If you cannot hold the foot unaided, use your towel to catch the foot. Reach down to the foot (or along the towel) so that the back bends a little. The stretch is achieved by holding the foot (or the towel) *with a straight arm*, and slowly *straightening* the back—this action transfers the bend of the back to the back of the leg as a stretch. The direction to 'hold with a straight arm' is to ensure that any straightening action of the back is transferred to the hamstring muscles at the back of the leg, and also because it is easier to hold the final stretch position for longer if the biceps muscles (the front of the upper arm) are not being used. The straightening action is also an isometric strengthening exercise for the back muscles running the whole length of the spine. *Do not compromise straightness in the back to get the body closer to the leg.* Hold the final position for ten breaths in and out. An even longer stay in this position yields good results—the hamstrings are powerful muscles, often very tight, and respond well to a long stretch.

The second photograph shows the position a partner adopts to assist in this movement. My partner is supporting my back where it was bending the most. A contraction can be done in this position too, if you are careful. Once supported in the starting position (whether using a towel or not) check to ensure that your back is straight. If it is, gently press back against your partner *using the muscles of the back of the leg* for five to ten seconds. Relax, re-straighten the back, and bend further forwards, from the hip. Let your partner support the final position for a minimum of ten breaths.

See a version of exercise 27 (pp. 88–89) which reduces the involvement of the back muscles to a minimum, and may be more comfortable for some people.

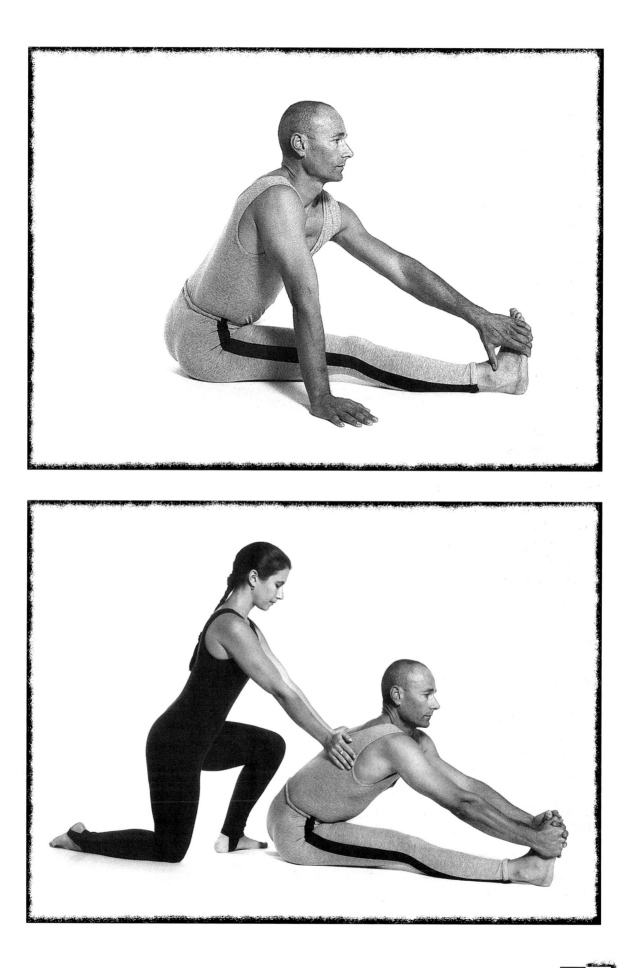

20. *Iliopsoas (part of* salute to sun) *with partner; C–R*

This version of the hip flexor stretch is far more effective than the solo version outlined in chapter one. The advantages of using this version are twofold: the subtle positioning required to stretch these muscles effectively is easier to achieve with a partner, and the use of the contraction component focuses the stretch even more closely on the hip flexors (deactivation of the stretch reflex by doing work at the end of the normal range of movement).

Positioning of the hips with respect to the line of the legs is critical. The most common fault in the performance of this movement is that as the hips move forward and down towards the floor, the hip of the back leg lags behind (due to tightness in the very muscles we want to stretch) and, in relative terms, rotates in the opposite direction to the main movement. As this happens, the stretch is moved from *iliopsoas* to the *quadriceps* group (front thigh muscles), thereby rendering the stretch ineffective.

Look at the photographs. Assume the starting position (front foot well in front of knee, back leg back, weight on knee). It is desirable to have the back leg's knee on a padded surface to avoid any discomfort to the kneecap. Ask your partner to take a hook grip on the hip bone of the front leg, and press on the hip of the back leg, behind the hip joint on the bottom itself, as shown. This hooking and pressing force induces a rotation into your hips which will counter the tendency for you to lose the stretch in the place you want it. With your hips held in position (with the back hip at least level with the other, and ideally forward, as might be seen from above), let both hips move forward and down. Have your partner *maintain* the alignment of both hips by maintaining the rotation force (pressing the back leg's hip forward). Sink down as far as you can, until the desired stretch is felt. Hold this stretch for a few breaths in and out.

Once in the full stretch position, the contraction is achieved by you trying to bring the back leg forward gently. Your partner will have to increase the pressing effort on the back hip slightly to counter the additional rotational force produced by your efforts. Hold the

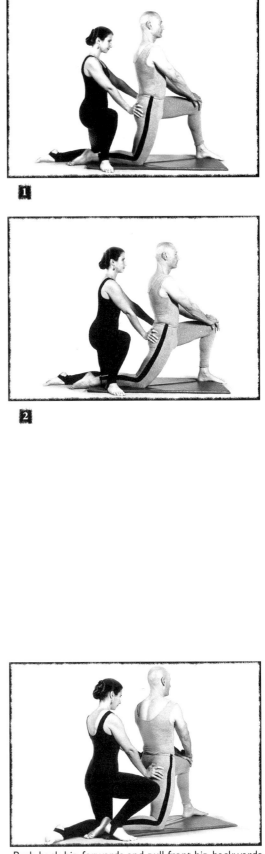

1

2

Push back hip forwards and pull front hip backwards

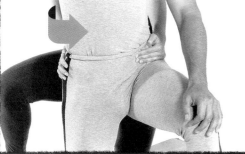

1

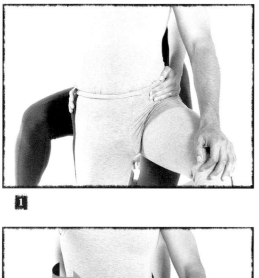

2 Press your back hip forwards

contraction for six to ten seconds. Relax, take in a deep breath and, as you breathe out, let the hips (still maintained in the correct position) go a little further to the floor. Hold the final stretched position for ten breaths. Repeat for the other leg. Critically compare right with left.

Check your form. If the lower back hyperextends strongly, resulting in an obvious curve backwards, you will need to provide an additional counteracting force. This is done by pressing down on the front knee with your support hand and tightening the abdominal muscles. This will tilt the top of the pelvis backwards and reduce the arch in the back. If you do this, you will immediately feel an increase in the stretch in the front of the back leg. For the same reason, you must not lean forwards over the front leg. This avoids the stretch by letting the pelvis tilt forwards.

If one side is tighter than the other, begin with the tight side in your next stretching session, then stretch the looser side, and re-stretch the tight side once again. In time, you will be able to bring the function of both sides nearer a balance.

For some people, the muscles you are trying to stretch become apparent only when they try to bring the back leg forward in the stretch. Retention of the alignment of the hips is critical to the success of the exercise.

If you find balancing in the pose difficult, check the width of placement of your front foot and your supporting knee; you will need hip width or slightly wider. You and your partner may use a wall against the front leg side of your body for stability also. Alternatively, because you do not need to press your back leg's hip forwards yourself when assisted, place a chair on this side of the body and use your hand to support yourself. The efficacy of the pose will be reduced if you are concentrating on balancing.

21. Hip/buttock (part of salute to the sun)

The start position is similar to the last exercise, but here the focus is the complex of hip/lower back muscles of the front leg. Support yourself on both hands, placed on the inside of the front leg. Place the foot in front of the knee for support. If you find it difficult to take this position, support yourself on a low box or similar object. Taking the weight of your body on your hands, slowly straighten the back leg (or get it as close to straight as you can). Look to the front (the action of looking forward straightens the upper back). Pull back on your hands a little without letting them slip along the floor (this action will help to straighten the lower back). Holding the back as straight as possible, let the arms bend until you feel a stretch in the bottom muscles. Let yourself go only as far forward as you can while maintaining a straight back. Do not let the hip of the back leg sink to the floor—the hips need to remain level for best effects. Hold for a few breaths in and out. To this point, you will have confined the stretch to part of the hamstring muscles (long head of *biceps femoris*), the bottom muscle (*gluteus maximus*), and perhaps the adductor muscles if they are tight. See the illustration for details.

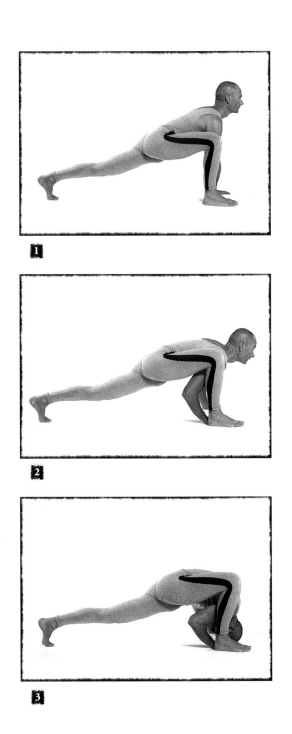

The next part of the movement stretches the muscles of the lower back as well. Take a breath in, check that the hips are level, and as you breathe out, let the arms bend further and also let the head go forward until the lower back is stretched too. Hold the final position for a few breaths in and out. This position is strenuous, and the supporting arms will be working hard. To come out of the position, always take a breath in and hold it in until you stand up. This will reduce the tendency to feel light headed—always a possibility when doing a difficult movement with the head lower than the heart. Rest for a moment or two before stretching the other side.

The reason the hamstring muscles are not emphasised in this movement (except as described) is because the knee is flexed. Assuming that you can maintain good form to this point, you can increase the stretch in the hamstring muscles in a second stretch by relaxing, moving the front foot further forward (with respect to the knee), and restretching. Placing the foot further forward increases the stretch in the hamstrings. Do not be tempted to exaggerate the forward placement of the foot.

A C–R stretch can improve hip flexibility. In the final stretch position, try to press the front foot into the floor gently. This action engages the illustrated muscles. Hold the contraction for a few seconds and restretch, while holding the hips level to avoid the tendency for the hip of the straight leg to sink to the floor.

Right hip in the extended position showing stretched muscles

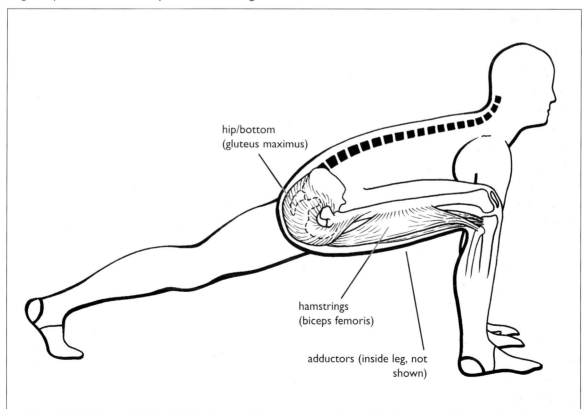

hip/bottom
(gluteus maximus)

hamstrings
(biceps femoris)

adductors (inside leg, not
shown)

22. Extension over support

So far, we have concentrated mainly on various forward bending and rotation movements. The recommendation often made for people suffering back pain to undertake backward bending exercises is not wise—the great majority of back pain sufferers find these movements painful. Thus the forward bending and rotation exercises should be used to relieve pain in the first instance. However, to return one's back to full function, extension movements are also required. Such exercises should be included in your routine only when the original pain has subsided to the point where your daily movements are comfortable and relatively pain free. Use your discretion—and if the inclusion of extension movements irritates the recovering back structures, discontinue them until the discomfort reduces, and cautiously begin adding them again.

The advantages of the first suggested extension position are that because it requires no strength for its support it can be held for a considerable length of time (letting you relax into the stretch), and because the body is prone and supported along its length, there is minimal compression on the vertebrae.

You will need a cylindrical firm pillow of suitable diameter, or a small and large firm cushion of sizes that will support about half the length of your back, or a little more. Place the small cushion on top of the larger one. Sit on the floor with your knees bent and with your back to the support. Use your arms to lower yourself over the support until you are lying across it. After the body is supported along its length, let the neck extend fully. This precaution will prevent the neck from being overextended. Rest in this position for a few breaths and, when comfortable and relaxed, slowly raise the arms backwards until they are stretched out overhead. This is the final position. Hold it for ten breaths or so. To return to the start position, bring the arms back to your side, place them on the floor, and use them to lift yourself up into the sitting position. While doing this, try to keep the rest of the body relaxed—in particular, do not use the groin or stomach muscles to return you to the sitting position. This direction is to avoid using the hip flexors (which attach to the anterior surfaces of the lumbar vertebrae) to sit up—doing so from this position

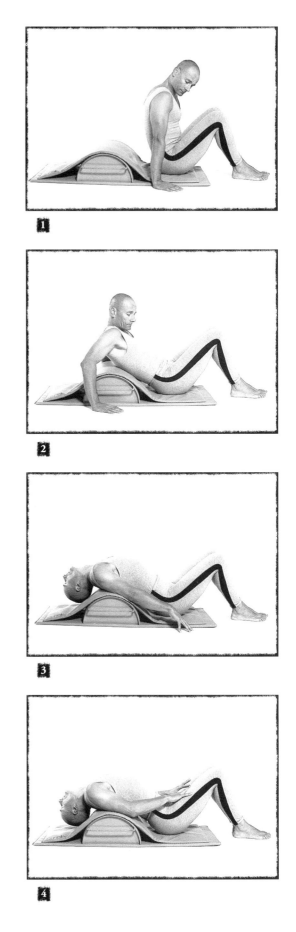

1

2

3

4

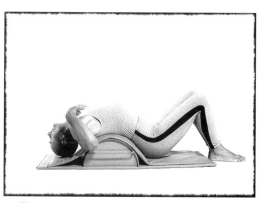

5

may make the lower back feel very uncomfortable. An alternative method of sitting up is to roll slowly to the side before getting up. Experiment with your position on the support. The last three photographs show a position emphasising the middle and lower back.

Assuming the exercise does not make the back feel worse, you may make the stretch stronger by using a higher support, or by slowly extending one leg at a time. When both legs are extended, breathe deeply and try to let the body relax completely.

When relaxed, you should feel the stretch in the abdominal area (the front of the body between the ribs and the hips), between the ribs and in the chest, too, when you raise the hands overhead. Regular practice of these kinds of movements will also help reduce the tendency for the upper back to bend forward and the shoulders hunch forward as you get older. These relatively passive extension movements prepare the body for the more difficult backwards bending poses.

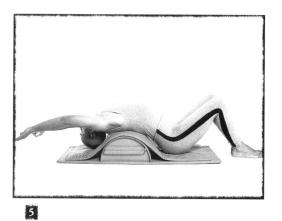

1

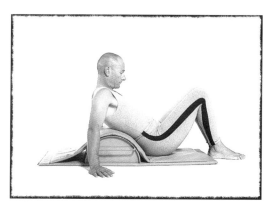

2

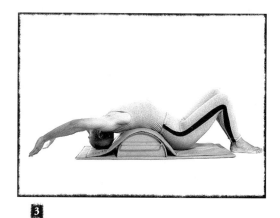

3

23. *Modified* cobra *pose; suspended version*

The next exercise is described in two forms, because one's proportion (lengths of body segments) substantially influences the final effects of the pose. The critical aspect of this pose is in keeping the lower back muscles completely relaxed while using only the arms to lift the shoulders and incline the upper body backwards.

This exercise, in various forms, has been a popular recommendation of physiotherapists. The underlying rationale is that if intervertebral disc material is bulging posteriorly, bending the spine backwards will 'push' or 'squeeze' the material back into place (through pressure from the bony structures of the vertebrae as they slide backwards over one another). The problem with this approach is that back-bending movements commonly irritate the back pain sufferer, probably through compression of the same joints. Such compression sensations will be exacerbated by any tension in the muscles running along the spine. For this reason exercises which relax these muscles should be used in the first instance, and back-bending movements should be added only when backward bending can be performed reasonably comfortably.

The conventional way to approach this stretch (the cobra pose in yoga) is to tense the bottom muscles before starting and to hold these muscles tight during the pose. The problem with this direction is that the untrained person almost always tenses the lower back muscles as well—the very thing we are trying to avoid.

The starting position is lying face-down, legs together, with your hands flat on the floor underneath the shoulders. If you think that you may not be particularly flexible backwards, place your hands further out to the *sides*, so that your shoulders will not be lifted quite as high when the arms are straightened. Deliberately relax the whole body. Take a deep breath in, and as you begin to breathe out, use only the arm muscles to elevate the upper body slowly, leaving the front of the hips on the floor. Use your partner to monitor any tightening of the lower back muscles, by asking them to place a hand on these muscles just above the bottom. As soon as any significant tightening is detected, lower yourself a fraction, relax, and try again. If you can keep these lower

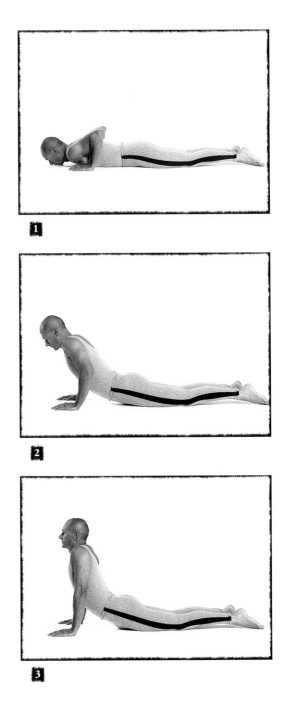

1

2

3

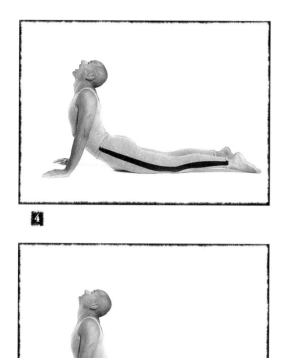

4

5

back muscles relaxed, this exercise is an effective and comfortable stretch for the front of the body.

As soon as you have reached maximum arm extension, pause and breathe in and out a few times, trying to keep the body as relaxed as possible. Breathe in, and draw the shoulders as far back as you can. Be careful that this action does not tense the muscles along the spine. If it does, concentrate on the first part of the exercise only. Hold the final position for five breaths.

Once comfortable in the final position, the stretch may be enhanced by opening the mouth and tilting the head back. Once the head is back, slowly close the mouth. Hold this position for a few breaths in and out.

The recovery position is shown in the final photograph overleaf.

A variation is referred to as the 'suspended' version. Begin in the push-up position—the body's weight supported on straight arms and on the balls of the feet, with the body held straight. Look at the photographs. Lower yourself into the stretch position by letting the body relax and by letting the body's weight bring the hips towards the floor. The only parts of the body exerting any force should be the muscles at the back of the arms, used to keep the arms straight. On no account should the back muscles be tight—rather, let them go completely slack and slowly let gravity bring the hips to the floor. Notice that the body sinks between the shoulders too (this requires that the muscles of the trunk, including the muscles under the arms, be relaxed). As soon as the front of the legs touch the floor, carefully straighten them so that you are suspended between hands and feet. The head should be in the neutral position at this point. Providing the lower back feels comfortable, cautiously bring the shoulders back. This instruction is given because this action tends to tighten the lower back muscles, which we do not want. If this happens to you, re-do the pose without this last action. Rest in the final form of the movement for at least five breaths in and out.

Always finish this pose (either version) by coming out of it slowly and immediately rolling over onto your back and clasping the bent knees to the chest. This action will gently stretch the lower back muscles, which usually (despite one's best efforts) will have tightened up a little during the pose. Hold the knees to the chest until the lower back feels relaxed (see the last photograph in the sequence). Any of the forward bending exercises (like the chair movements) can be substituted for the knees to the chest movement if you prefer.

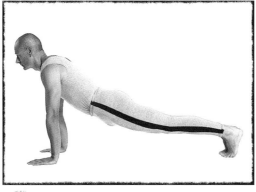

1

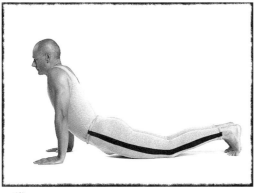

2

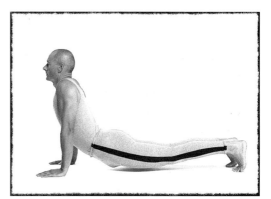

3

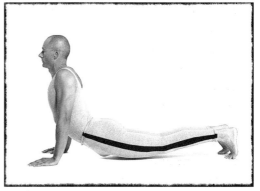

4

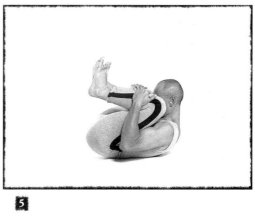

5

24. Quadriceps: standing; lying; C–R

If the hip flexor exercise (the *iliopsoas* stretch above) is difficult for you, you may include a stretch that affects the *quadriceps*, the large muscles of the front of the thighs, as these muscles are likely to be tight too. Three quadriceps stretches are offered here, and any is a suitable warm-up movement for the hip flexor stretch.

Try the standing version first. This is slightly different to the lying version, as some extension of the leg is possible (with respect to the pelvis), and accordingly the top part of the thigh will be stretched in addition to the middle and lower sections. Stand opposite a wall as shown for balance, and lift the foot as close to the bottom as possible, and then clasp the ankle. If you wish to stretch the instep as well, hold the toes. Bring the foot as close to the bottom as possible, and stand up straight. If you cannot hold the leg (through tightness in the thigh), you can place the foot on a chair behind you (placed in such a way as to be stable), and stretch the thigh by shuffling back towards the chair.

A partner can assist here, by placing one hand on the foot next to the bottom (pressing the foot closer), clasping the other hand around the knee of the bent leg, and gently pulling the knee back. The pulling movement should have the first hand as its axis; that is, the first hand fixes the position of the foot and the hip forward, and the other pulls the knee into the extension position. Two different contractions are possible. The first is an attempt to straighten the held leg (for the usual six to ten seconds). The second is trying to pull the folded leg away from the partner (towards the wall) for the same duration. The partner enhances the stretch by pressing the foot closer to your bottom, or by pulling the folded leg further in extension, or both. These C–R stretches may be done separately if the resulting stretch is too strong. Repeat for the other leg.

Jennifer is demonstrating a third version of the *quadriceps* stretch. Because you can control the degree of knee flexion by how close you take the hips to the wall, this version will be more comfortable in the knees for some people than the versions shown overleaf. Place a cushion or mat under the supporting knee. Ease the calf muscle of the leg against the wall out of the way (as shown overleaf), and move the hips backwards to feel the stretch. If you have a tendency to hyperextend in the lower back (very likely if *iliopsoas* are tight), press both hands down on the knee of the front leg as shown, and tighten the abdominal muscles. This action pulls the front of the pelvis upwards, flattens the lumbar spine and increases the stretch in the thigh muscle. Hold the body vertical and bring the body closer to the wall to increase the stretch.

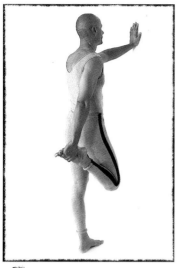

1

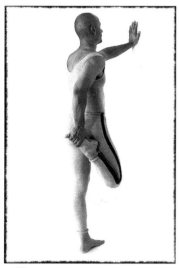

2

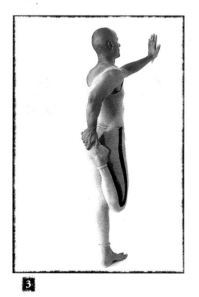

3

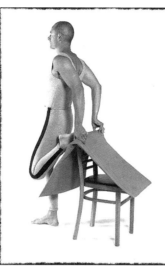

An easier version

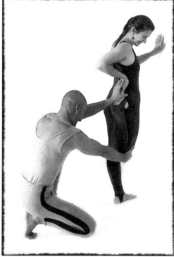

1

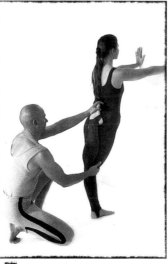

2

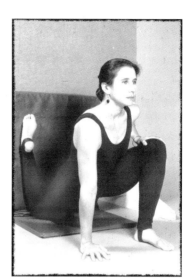

1

2

The seated version of the thigh stretch has the advantage of being easier to hold for more extended periods. Look at the photograph. When getting into this position, always push the calf muscle *out of the way* before bringing the foot close to the leg. (Both the calf and hamstring muscles, if tight, resist flowing out of the way in this position, and if this is the case the bulk of the muscles tends to force the knee joint apart. This tendency is exacerbated by exercising in pants that are too tight, or that do not stretch.) You must be able to sit with this buttock on the ground. If you cannot, place a firm cushion under the hip of the straight leg so that the hips remain level. The thicker the support, the less the stretch in the thigh. There should be no discomfort in the knee of the folded leg. The knees should stay close together, and the foot of the folded leg should point directly backwards.

Assuming that the position attained so far is comfortable, lean back onto the hands, then the elbows, to increase the stretch. Under no circumstances must you let the lower back hyperextend—if in doubt, tense the abdominal muscles and curl the body forwards. (Recall the remarks made about the *iliopsoas* muscles. These are stretched in this position, and if tight will pull the lumbar spine forward and hyperextend the back, which can be painful.)

To help stabilise the final position, and to help to tilt the body's weight in the direction of the hip of the bent leg, you may bend the other leg and place the foot flat on the floor near the bottom, and grasp its ankle to hold it there. Refer to the accompanying photographs. This action makes holding the final position more comfortable and increases the stretch because the hips are held level. Lying in this way makes it more difficult to avoid the stretch in the folded leg, and the form is better preserved. This assistance technique may be used in the intermediate positions too, for increased effect. Hold the final position for at least ten normally-paced breaths in and out.

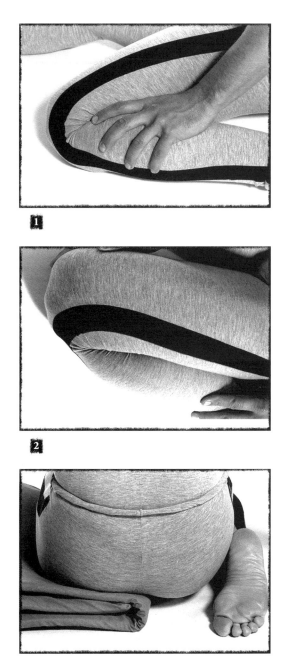

If you cannot sit with both buttocks on the ground

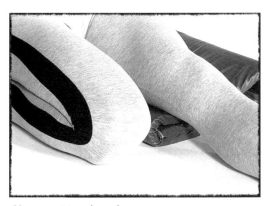

Above position, from front

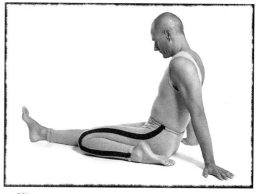

1

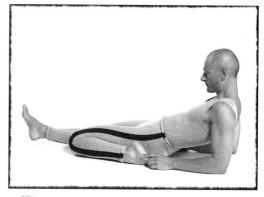

2

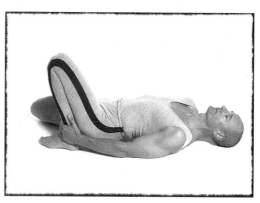

Hold ankle for support, and to keep hips level

25. Half-bridge

The ease of doing this exercise depends largely on your proportion, especially the length of the arms in relation to the length of the upper body. Try it gently, but do not be discouraged if you cannot do it—it only suits some bodies.

Caution: those with problems that restrict forward bending of the neck should avoid this movement, as the neck is strongly bent forward if you can attain the final position. This aspect may be reduced by placing mats under the *shoulders* and letting the head rest lower on the floor, so that in the final position the neck will be less stretched. Detail is shown later, in the exercise called *modified plough pose*, the second-last exercise in this chapter.

Hold the ankles with a hook grip as shown, because this generally permits a firmer hold. (Note that a 'hook' grip uses the whole hand to hold the ankle rather than thumb and fingers in opposition as is usual). Strongly tighten the bottom muscles and, pushing from the hips, lift the body off the floor as far as you can. Push *only* with the hips. In particular, do not try to increase the bend in the upper body by arching the back muscles. When you have lifted the hips as high as possible, gently try to straighten the legs to complete the position. This last action pulls the upper body into a backward curve. As a backward bending movement, there is relatively little compression in the lumbar spine, and compared to other backwards bending exercises, there is a stronger feeling of a stretch in the front of the body, especially in the chest and shoulders. Hold the final position for at least a few breaths. Let yourself down onto the floor, and immediately curl up clasping the knees to the chest.

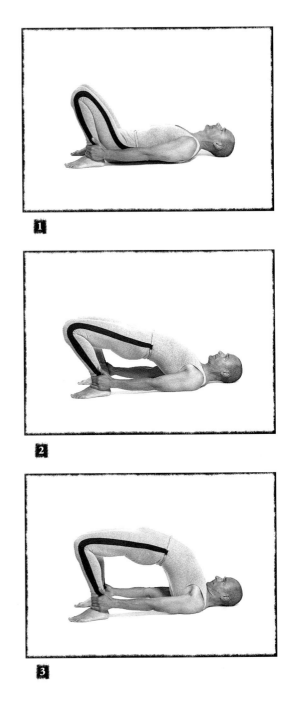

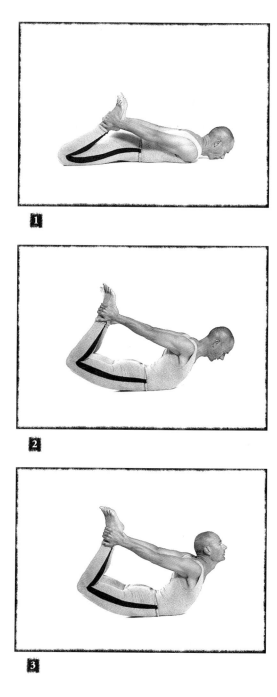

1

2

3

26. *Modified* locust *pose*

In some ways similar to the previous pose is the *locust* pose from yoga. One advantage of the locust pose is that most people can achieve the starting position because the feet are closer to the hands, whereas one's proportion can make the half-bridge difficult to get into. However, one disadvantage of the locust pose is that there is considerable pressure on the abdominal area which some people will find uncomfortable.

Lie on your stomach, reach back and grasp each leg, one at a time. Lift both the chest and the thighs off the ground, not by arching the back, but by gently tensing the thighs. Visualise drawing a bow—try to do so by trying to straighten the legs. A strong towel looped around the feet permits an easier version. As you try to straighten the legs, lift the head, and *by trying to straighten the legs*, let the body be stretched upwards and backwards. Breathing will be difficult due to the weight on the abdomen and the stretched position, but try to hold the final shape for ten breaths in and out, in as normal a fashion as you can manage. *Under no circumstances hold your breath.* When you lower yourself to the floor, immediately roll face up and clasp the knees to the chest for a breath or two, to relax the back muscles, as with the other back bending movements.

27. Single hamstring, seated, with partner, lying; C–R

This exercise allows you to concentrate your attention on the hamstring muscles of one leg at a time. The advantage of this is that the entire strength of the trunk muscles can be used to maintain the straightness of the lower back, and the whole upper body can thus be used as a lever for stretching the hamstrings.

The three muscles of the hamstrings originate at the *ischial tuberosities* (the two bones we sit on) and run down the back of the thigh and cross the knee joint to finish at the lower leg. For this reason, the leg needs to be straight to stretch these muscles completely. See the illustration for details.

Sit as shown. If you think that you may not be able to reach a foot with both hands easily, loop a towel or something similar around the foot and hold with both hands. Allow the back to bend a little to find the starting position. Once the foot is held, arch the whole back backwards—it is the straightening action which stretches the hamstrings, by tilting the top of the pelvis forwards. The straightening effort also helps to strengthen the back muscles (by isometric contraction). You may need to ask your partner if your back is straight, as it is a difficult thing for most beginners to feel.

The easiest of the assistance exercises is to have your partner support whichever part of your back wants to bend first as you increase the pulling effort on the foot. If your partner places his or her hands on this most curved part of the back, straightening the back (and holding the final stretch position) will require far less effort. You will also be able to hold the final position longer. Ensure that you look forwards and try to keep the chest lifted up. These directions will help keep the back straight.

The next most effective form of the exercise is to perform a contraction yourself, without support. This can be useful if you are stretching solo. This technique is most effective in preparing for holding a long static stretch. Assuming you are in the final stretch position, check to see if your back is straight (particularly the **lowest** part of the back—there should be a straight line from sacrum to neck). Pull back gently on the hands as

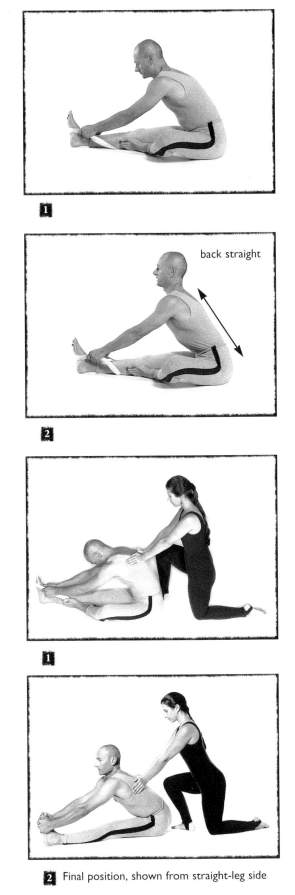

1

2 back straight

1

2 Final position, shown from straight-leg side

though you were trying to pull the hands and body away from the feet. If your form is correct, the only place you will feel any effort is in the hamstring muscles. If you feel the effort in your back, check its straightness and begin again. After holding the contraction for six to ten seconds, relax completely, breathe in deeply and as you breathe out pull yourself forward slowly (holding the chest up as shown) until the required stretch is felt. Hold the final position for at least ten breaths. Repeat for the other leg.

The muscles of the back of the leg

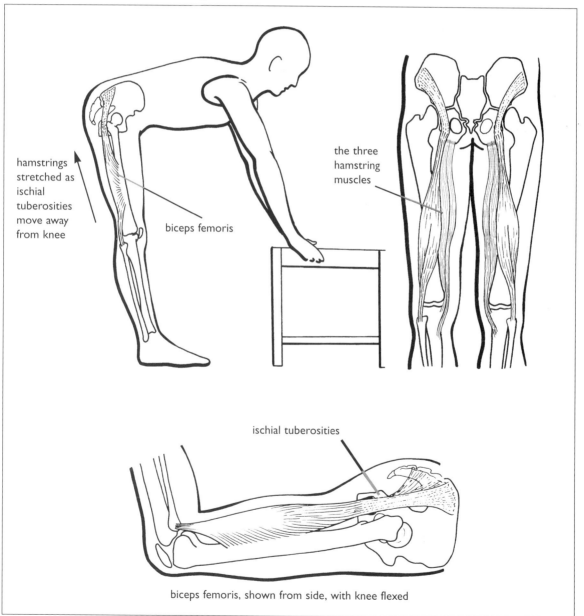

hamstrings stretched as ischial tuberosities move away from knee

biceps femoris

the three hamstring muscles

ischial tuberosities

biceps femoris, shown from side, with knee flexed

The most effective stretch for the hamstring muscles is the partner C–R stretch. This version of the exercise is recommended even if your hamstring muscles are particularly tight, because the positioning of the body ensures that there is no lower back involvement. Because the exercise is performed in the lying position, it is also relatively easy for both you and your partner to hold the final position. The stretch may be felt anywhere between the bottom and the calf muscle on the stretched leg.

Lie face up as shown. Have your partner sit on one of your outstretched legs (but not on the kneecap) and lift the other until you feel a gentle stretch along its length. Note how the partner must be in a position that permits relaxed and secure support of the lifted leg. Once in position, press the top leg (the one being held) directly down to the floor using the muscles at the back of the leg, for six to ten seconds. Do not press too hard the first time you try the movement—a third of your strength is about right. Stop pressing, relax completely and take a deep breath. As you breathe out ask your partner to lift the leg *very slowly* higher until you feel the required stretch. The leg should remain straight (not bent to avoid the stretch), so your partner may need to apply a straightening effort above the knee as shown—this is preferable to you expending energy to hold the leg straight yourself. Relax completely in the stretched position, letting your partner do all the work of holding the leg. Imagine the muscles in which you feel the stretch lengthening and relaxing as you breathe, particularly each breath out. Hold the final position for at least ten breaths, and repeat for the other leg. If you push the leg down in the direction of the floor while holding it straight as suggested, *biceps femoris* will usually do most of the work. This is where most of the stretching effect will be felt, individual variations notwithstanding.

You may wish to try an alternative hamstring C–R stretch to determine which of the two is more effective for you. Assume the same starting position, but instead of pushing the leg to the floor, use the muscles at the back of the leg to try to flex the leg at the knee (that is, try to pull the heel back to the bottom). Let your partner stretch the leg further up as before. This action engages

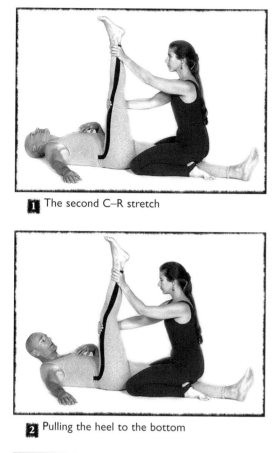

1 The second C–R stretch

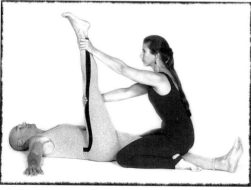

2 Pulling the heel to the bottom

3

the bulk of the hamstring group, and for some people may prove the better stretch. Both versions should be attempted, and for the best effect, do one after the other. Hook first, then press the whole leg back, relax, and let your partner stretch you. The contractions, relaxation, and re-stretch sequence may be repeated for further effect. Always hold the final position for a minimum of ten breaths. *If you cannot, you are overdoing the stretch.*

In either case, the action of stretching the leg further away from the floor also stretches the sciatic nerve, which is often involved in back pain. The sciatic nerve is the longest nerve in the body, and its significance is discussed in some detail below. Consider the final stretch position, and look at the position of the foot in relation to the leg. A strongly pointed foot suggests a shortening of the calf muscles. If you see this, you can intensify the stretch by asking your partner to apply weight to the ball of the foot to increase the flexion at the ankle. This action can use a C–R stretch effectively. Press the ball of the foot back against your partner's resistance, and restretch. Always do these stretches separately before doing them in sequence. A strongly flexed ankle in the final position of the hamstring stretch is also a maximum stretch for the sciatic nerve.

28. Standing calf (sciatic nerve)

Another exercise with beneficial effects on the sciatic nerve is one that specifically stretches the calf muscles. If sciatica is a problem for you, you should include this exercise in your routine. Whereas the previous exercise derived its effect on the sciatic nerve from flexion of both the hip and ankle joints, this exercise concentrates on the ankle.

Place yourself facing a wall as shown. The front foot is used for stability only, and plays no other part in the stretch. Support yourself on outstretched hands while bent forward at the hips with the back held straight. Place the back foot a metre or more away from the wall. If supporting yourself on your arms is too tiring, you can rest on the elbows and forearms instead with no loss of effect on the ankle. Press the back leg straight (necessary to stretch the top calf muscle, *gastrocnemius*). While holding the heel firmly on the floor, move the hips towards the wall until you feel sufficient stretch. Each calf muscle supports at least our whole body's weight daily, and is often resistant to being stretched, so hold the final stretch for a minimum of ten breath cycles.

It is essential that the foot of the leg being stretched is directly in front of the shin. It is a common mistake in this exercise to permit the ankle to pronate (roll inwards). Pronating avoids the proper stretch, and places an unsymmetrical stretching force on the Achilles tendon, which (potentially) could be dangerous. If you have a tendency to do this, press a little extra weight onto the outside (little toe side) of the foot, and keep an eye on the shape of the ankle.

A contraction used here can help loosen the calf muscle. Once in the stretch position, gently press the ball of the foot into the floor for five seconds or so. Relax, breathe in, and on an exhalation, press the heel to the floor and take the hips a little closer to the wall. This is a strong stretch. Hold the final position for ten breaths.

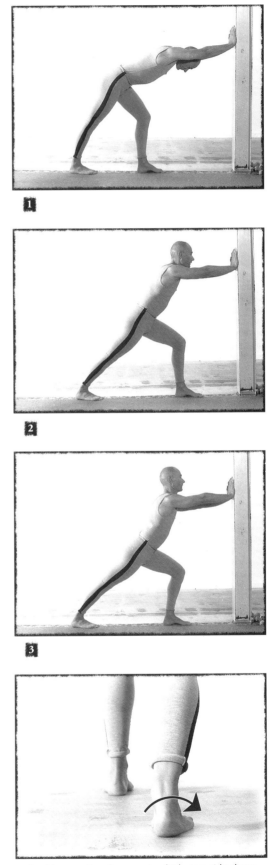

Avoid pronation, by pressing little toe side down

Sciatic nerve, and muscles of the lower leg

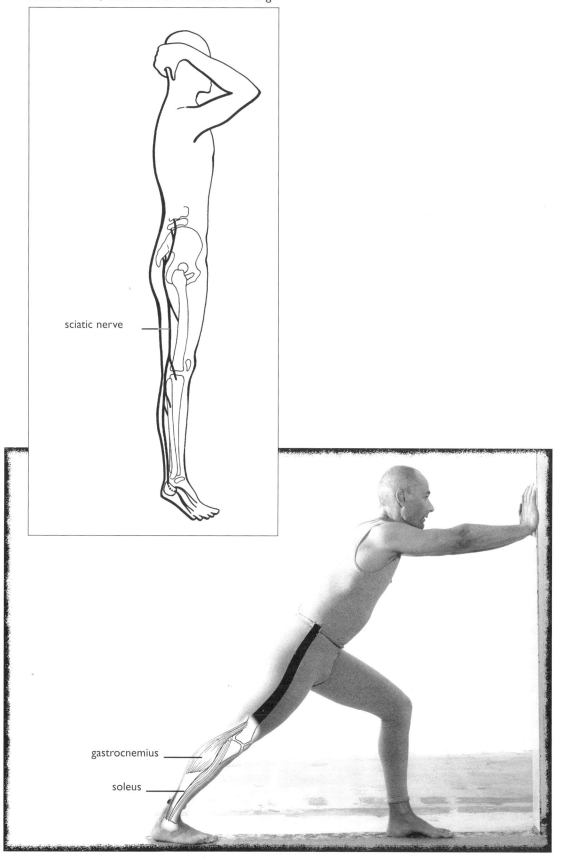

sciatic nerve

gastrocnemius

soleus

29. *One-leg* dog *pose*

One of the strongest stretches for the sciatic nerve, calf and hamstring muscles combined is a modified yoga pose, the *dog* pose. The exercise presented here is a modified 'one-legged' version, which has a number of advantages over the traditional pose. One advantage is that, because only one leg is being stretched, all the muscles of the trunk can be used to maintain straightness in the spine. Another is that the weight of the body will stretch one leg further than two (effectively double the weight, so double the stretching force).

The instruction regarding alignment of the foot with the leg being stretched applies here too. To begin, press the heel of the leg to be stretched to the floor, and hold it there. Place your hands on a suitable support; that is, one that will not move away from you under horizontal forces. A low chair or couch anchored against a wall is ideal. If you are sufficiently flexible, bend at the waist, and place the hands on the floor. Walk your hands away from you, holding the heel on the ground. The other leg will be tucked behind you or, if you prefer, placed in front with the knee flexed (as in the previous exercise which used the wall for support). The latter approach gives you greater control over the final stretch. Stretch each leg in turn, for a minimum of ten breaths.

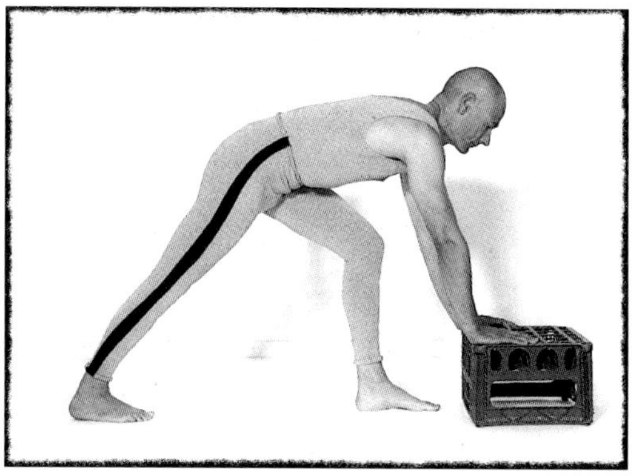

Place the support against a wall to ensure that it does not slide away from you

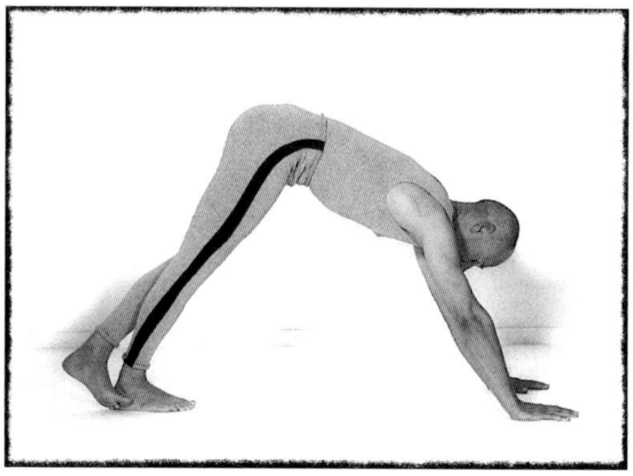

1

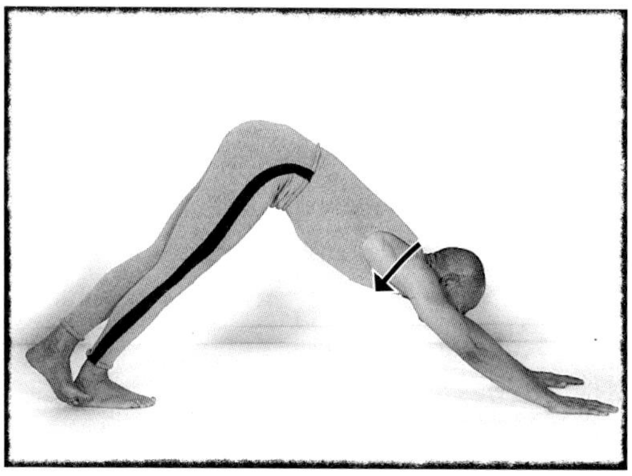

2

30. Standing lateral flexion; roll out

Using a wall in this movement ensures correct alignment and provides support. The aim is to stretch all of the side waist muscles, the obliques, in the first instance. As these become more flexible, the exercise will also stretch one half of the *quadratus lumborum* pair and half of the deep spinal muscles, which may be involved in back pain. The abductors of the leg will also be stretched, including the far end (that is, the distal end, in this case towards the knee) of *tensor fascia lata*. Compare left lateral flexion with right—symmetry is desirable in this movement.

Standing with the weight evenly on both feet, lean the body against the wall, feeling contact at the heels, back of the knees (or calf muscles), the bottom, the back of the shoulders, and the head. Use a chair off to one side for assistance if you feel vulnerable (too extended, or not sufficiently supported) in the movement. Try to maintain the relationship of the shoulders to the pelvis. This is best done by maintaining shoulder and bottom contact with the wall. Lean to one side as shown, supporting yourself with one hand against the leg. If you feel that you are going too far, you can stop yourself with this hand. When you have leant as far to one side as you can comfortably, grasp the leg with this hand. Two hand positions are shown—choose the one that gives you the best support. Leaning on this hand, reach the other arm out and over the head as far as you can—the locus of the stretch will extend from a local area above the hip you are stretching to the whole of that side. Hold the final position for five breaths only.

To come out of the stretch, do *not* reverse the actions you used to get into it. Instead, very slowly roll the top shoulder away from the wall, trying to increase the sidewards stretch all the while. As you rotate the shoulder forward, your apparent flexibility at the waist will increase noticeably, and you will need to increase the lean to the side just to maintain the stretch sensation. The locus of the stretch will move too, from just above the hip to further towards the spine itself as the shoulder rotates forward. If you find a position that feels particularly good in this transition, pause there for a breath or two. Repeat for the other side.

Schematic of hip muscles affected

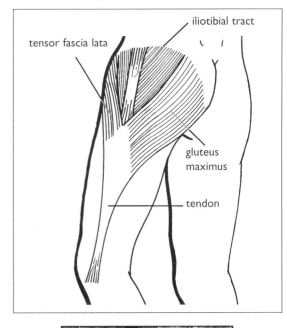

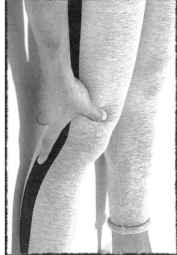

You must be able to *lean* on the support hand

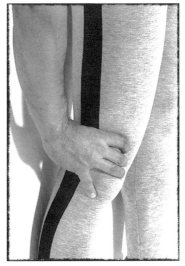

Alternative grip, better for thicker legs

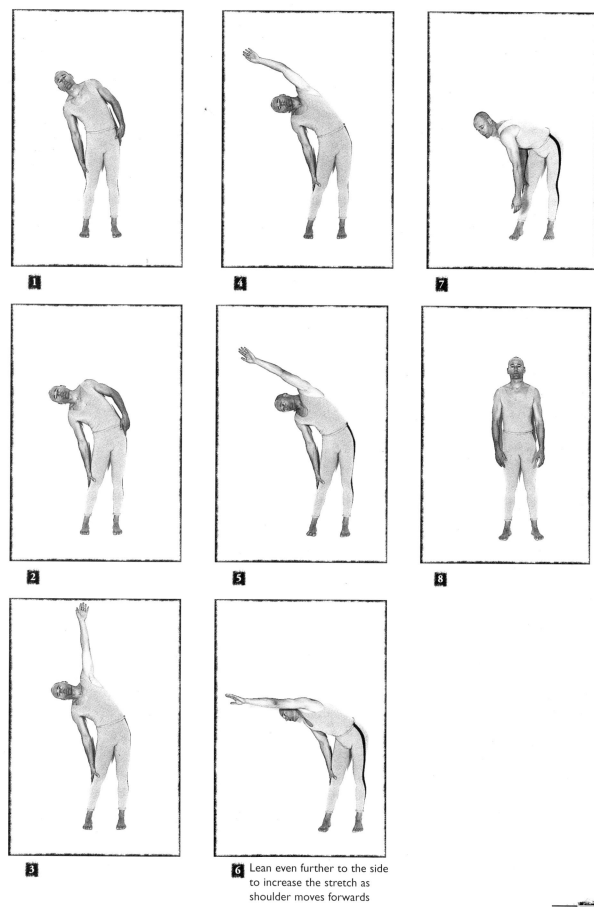

1

2

3

4

5

6 Lean even further to the side
to increase the stretch as
shoulder moves forwards

7

8

31. Lying side stretch (suspended)

The previous stretch may be too strong if your back is sensitive. Bending to the side while standing requires the facet joints of the lumbar spine to slide over each other and, under compression, pain may result. This exercise removes much of this load, but requires careful positioning and some strength in the arms for support. The main effect of this exercise is on the hip abductors. This exercise may be useful for those who are tight in this area—broadly speaking, from the lower back to mid-thigh, as occurs frequently in runners. The wall may also be used to maintain alignment in this version.

There are two ways of getting into the position shown. The first (requiring more arm strength but permitting more control) is to lie on the floor on one side with hips, legs, and shoulders against the wall. Place the hands as shown, and achieve the required stretch by pushing the hands away from the body, raising the body without letting the hip leave the floor. The arm of the shoulder furthest from the hips will do most of the work. If comfortable, you may use the waist muscles of the side you are bending towards to assist the lifting movement. The top leg may be bent and placed in front of the other for stability. If you use the top waist muscles for assistance, be sure to relax the muscles, by repeating the stretch briefly on the side you begin with after doing the second side. Roll the hip forwards and backwards a little to find the most effective stretch.

The second way begins by resting on the outstretched arm with the body held straight, as shown. The foot of the top hip's leg is used for support in front. As before, a wall may be used behind you to maintain alignment. Slowly let the body bend at the waist until you feel the required stretch. Rest in this position for five breaths or so. Repeat for the other side.

If you do not get sufficient stretch from this approach (it may be, for example, that you have relatively short arms and a long trunk) you may intensify the effect by resting your supporting hand on a block or similar object. Alternatively, the supporting foot may be rested on the block. Using a block under the hand tends to concentrate the stretch above the waist. Conversely, a block under the foot tends to move the point of maximum stretch below the hip joint. Experiment and

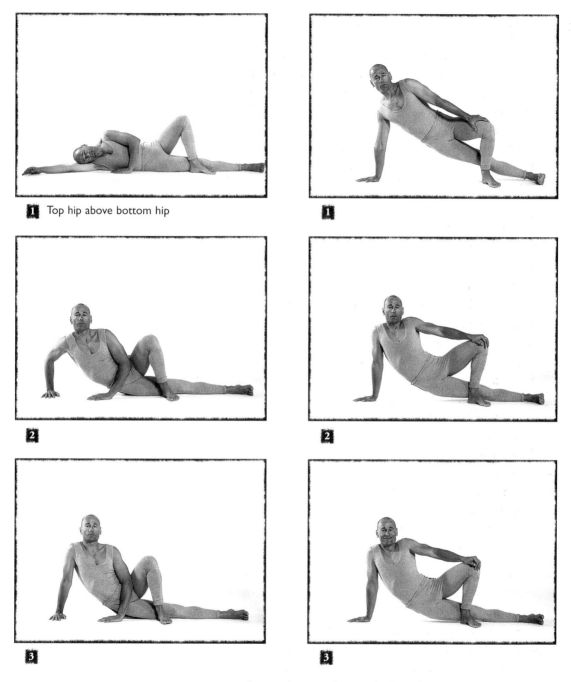

1 Top hip above bottom hip

1

2

2

3

3

choose the one that works best for you.

As shown, with the top hip directly over the bottom hip, the stretch will be felt on the outside of, and above, the bottom hip. To move the stretch *forwards,* roll the top hip forwards by walking the foot of the bent leg forwards; similarly, to move the stretch on the bottom hip backwards, roll the top hip backwards. In this way, the exercise can stretch a great number of hip and lower back muscles. Make these movements small, as even tiny movements can change which muscles will be affected.

32. Standing hamstring/lower back

On first examination this movement may appear to be merely the old 'touch-the-toes', but it is not. Physiotherapists and similar people working in rehabilitation have long recommended that stretching the hamstring muscles has a beneficial effect on low back pain. This may well be true, but not for the reasons usually given. Poor execution of the exercise—characterised by a rounding of the lower back—is the main reason why it works. When done by people with poor hamstring flexibility, the lower back muscles are stretched and this effect gives the relief. There is the possibility that the stretching of the sciatic nerve that accompanies this movement (regardless of whether or not it is performed technically well) also contributes to the beneficial effect ascribed to it.

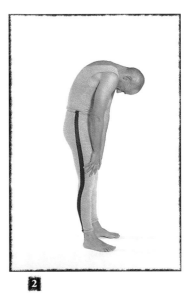

Done in the following way, the exercise can be, variously, a gentle lower back stretch, a gentle two-leg hamstring stretch, or a stronger one-leg hamstring stretch.

Begin by standing with your body's weight evenly distributed over both feet. Let the chin go as far forward as it can (rest it on the chest if comfortable). Let the upper back bend, followed by the middle and lower back. Let the whole back round out. Do these actions slowly, and if your back is at all sensitive, use your hands along the thighs and the shins to support yourself at all stages.

When you have bent as far forward as you can comfortably and if your back is not protesting, gently unweight the hands. Take the weight of the body off the hands gradually so that your body's weight comes onto the muscles of the back and back of legs. Let yourself hang there for five to ten breaths in and out. Be aware of where you feel the effects of what you are doing—the stretch may be felt along the back (or concentrated in a particular part) or anywhere from the bottom to the heels. Check that you are still dividing your weight evenly on both feet. If the stretch sensation is too strong—or if you are worried that it might become so—support yourself on a box or a low stool placed in front of your feet.

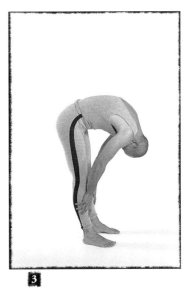

Now slowly let one leg flex slightly—just enough to take the stretch away from it, as shown. You will feel all the stretch in the straight leg. Hold this position for a few breaths. Now straighten the back a little to intensify the stretch in the leg. Hold this position for a few breaths.

To transfer the stretch to the other leg, slowly let the straight leg bend *before* straightening the first leg. Hold the stretch in the

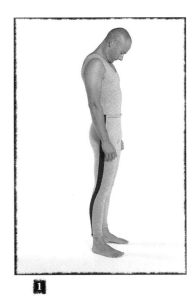

second leg for a few breaths. Compare left with right. If there is a difference (either in flexibility or perception of tightness or pain) restretch the tighter leg by bending the other and again straightening the one you want to stretch. Hold this final stretch for a few breaths also.

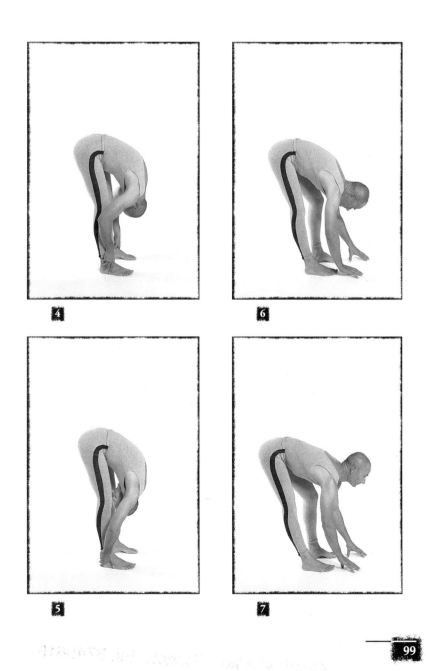

4

6

5

7

33. Isolation *return from standing flexion*

To return to the standing position, we will use an *isolation* exercise from dance. Yoga has a similar movement. The purpose here is both to return to the standing position, and to become more aware of how the back muscles work together. Although the thick muscles running up both sides of the spine appear to be quite large and continuous, they are composed of many small bundles of muscles spanning two, or several, vertebrae. Problem areas can be isolated quite precisely, and we can learn to move specific parts of the back.

To begin, bend both knees until the sensation of stretching the back of the legs has gone. At this point, the head and the body are hanging in a relaxed fashion from the hips. The purpose of the next series of movements is to learn to contract the muscles of the back, from top to bottom. To aid the process, visualise yourself slowly arching the body backwards, from the head all the way down the back to the hips, in sequence before you actually try the movement.

Slowly lift only the head up as far as you can. This activates mainly the muscles at the back of the neck. Now contract the muscles of the upper back. Next contract the middle back muscles. By this stage the back should be hollowed (concave posteriorly), and you should feel as though you are lifting yourself up, leading with the head. Imagine that there is a string attached to the top of your head and that you are being lifted up by it. Lastly, contract the muscles of the lower back. By this time the back will be as hollowed as you can make it, and the upper body will be making roughly a 45 degree angle with the floor. To complete the movement, stand up, still leading with the head.

If you repeat the movement a number of times, it will become more fluid and the sense of being able to isolate parts of the back will become stronger. Take note of any part of the back which moves as one section (that is, a section which does not permit isolation). Such a part will need further work.

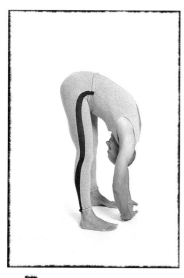

1

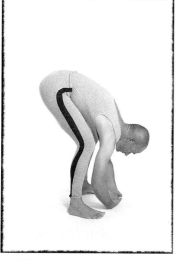

2

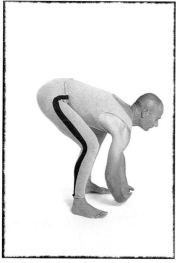

3

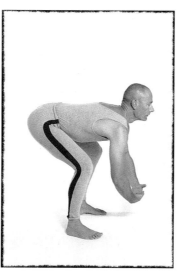

4

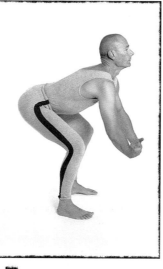

5

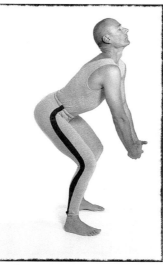

6

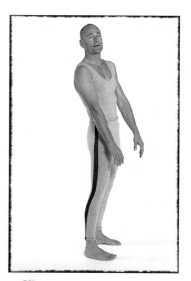

7

34. Upper back; chair, wall, floor version; C–R

Slumping of the shoulders and rounding of the upper back are common postural problems. Both these changes are extremely common phenomena accompanying ageing. A reduction in the suppleness of the muscles between the ribs (*intercostals*) and a shortening of the front arm muscles (*biceps*), the front shoulder muscles (*anterior deltoid*), and the chest muscles (*pectoralis major* and *minor*) are significant factors in these changes.

The role of these changes in neck pain is easy to visualise (and see). Any increased forward bending of the upper back results either in an increase in the curvature of the cervical spine (and possible increased compression of the facet joints) or the carrying of the head forward of its normal balanced position (requiring the posterior neck muscles to do more work to maintain posture in any position). Such extra work means that these muscles reach their work limit before they otherwise would. Here, work limit may be as simple as getting tired, or feeling noticeable tension.

Upper body muscles   Changes accompanying ageing

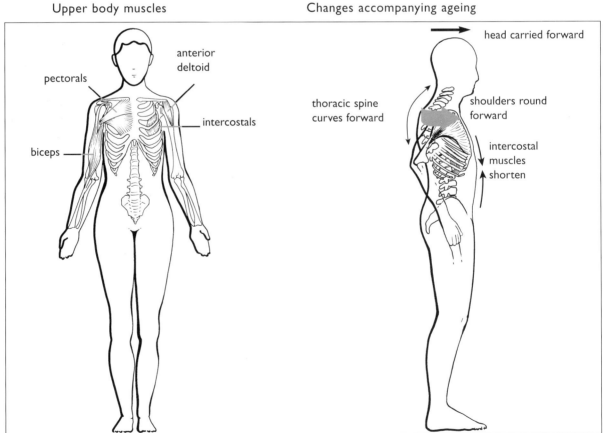

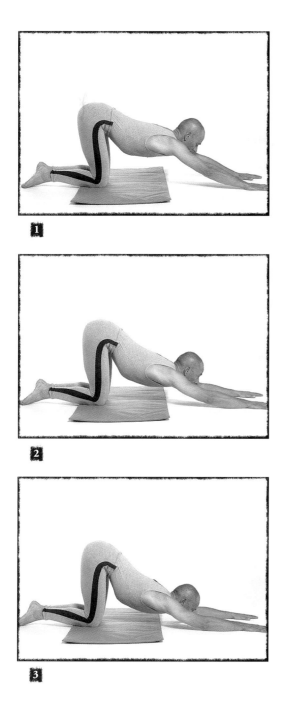

1

2

3

The role such changes may have in low back pain is less obvious. It is probably related to load redistribution necessitated by changes to the shape of the spine, and the additional strain placed on the lumbar vertebrae if the function of any other part of the spine is reduced. Whenever the head is carried forward of the centre of gravity, the muscles of the back are required to do additional work.

The purpose of the following poses (including the stronger partner C–R versions) is to 'open' the chest and increase the capacity of the middle and upper back to bend backwards. Open, used in this way, means to counter the normal (though undesirable) shortening of the muscles mentioned. After a period of practice, the shoulders will sit further back on the rib cage without conscious effort and the chest will appear and feel expanded.

The first version is both the least strenuous to hold and the most comfortable. You will need something to kneel on if you are working on a hard floor—a folded blanket is ideal. Kneel and walk yourself forward on your hands until the arms are fully extended in front of you at about shoulder width. Press the arms straight, extending them from the body as far as you can. Move forward on your hands until the hips are directly over the knees. Relax the legs. Look at the floor between your hands, take a deep breath, and on an exhalation let the upper body sink as close to the floor as it can. Keep the arms extended—the tendency will be to let the elbows bend and that will dissipate the effects of the pose. This is quite a subtle position and you will not derive the benefits until you let the body's own weight bring you closer to the floor. Hold the final position for ten to fifteen breaths in and out. To return to the starting position, bring your hands back to under the shoulders, come up to a hands and knees position, and fold the body over the legs. Rest in this final position for a few breaths.

A chair version can also be used, done in the office if you wish. Look at the accompanying photographs. This version is less strenuous, as the body's weight is supported by the chair. Place the chair at a distance from the wall which gives you the intensity of stretch you require. Look at a spot in between your hands. This will help initiate a bend backwards in the upper back by involving the *trapezius* muscles in the upper back. Here too, a partner can make the stretch more intense if desired, by placing his or her hand on the most forwards-curved part of the middle or upper back and applying a little weight.

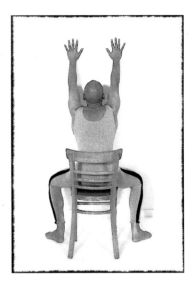

The next most intense version is the floor movement, with a partner. Consider the photographs. The partner is kneeling between my outstretched hands, with both hands placed on my upper back between my shoulder blades. The partner, as always, must be in a position that guarantees *stable* weight and permits quick removal of the applied weight if necessary. For this reason, the partner has her right foot forwards for stability. The partner does not *press* her weight, but rather *leans* her weight on me. Notice that her arm is about 90 degrees from the part of my back she is leaning on. Because of the shape of my back, this angle results in about half of her weight pressing down to the floor (extending the arms with respect to the body) and about half pressing back to my hips (helping the back to bend backwards).

Relax completely while keeping the arms pressed straight so that the upper body is pressed towards the floor. Hold the final position for five breaths. When being stretched in this position, it is essential that the partner does not lean too much weight on you. If you are tensing up against the weight it is probably too much.

If a stronger stretch is required, once in the final stretch position you may gently press your hands down onto the floor for about six seconds, using the whole body. This contracts all the muscles we are trying to stretch. With an exhalation, relax completely. You may need to ask your partner to lean a little more weight on you in the relaxed position to feel sufficient stretch. Hold the final position for five breaths in and out.

The last photograph shows a variation which may be used if the chest contacts the floor before the desired stretch is experienced. The elbows are placed on a rolled up mat or similar object. This version can be more comfortable in the shoulders for some people. Try all versions, and select the one that gives the best effects.

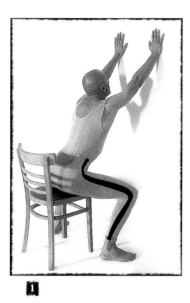

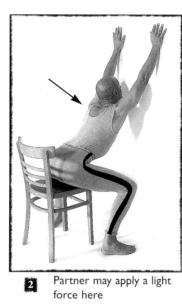

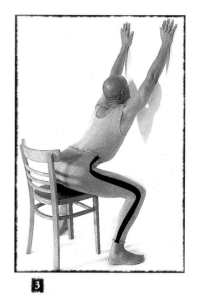

1

2 Partner may apply a light force here

3

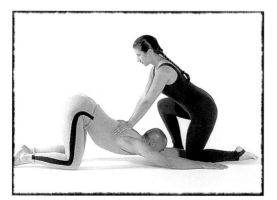

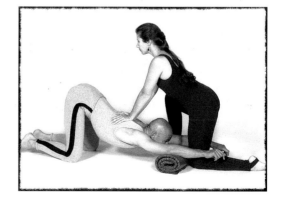

The standing version seems to stretch the muscles under the arms more than the floor version. Even done solo it is a much stronger stretch than the version above. Stand a metre or so away from a wall, facing it. Place the hands on the wall about half a metre above the shoulders. Bend the legs slightly to remove the hamstring stretching aspect and to remove compression from the lower back. Look up between your hands (this tenses the *trapezius* muscles and helps to extend the upper back). Press the arms out and away from the body as though you are trying to reach through the wall (this stretches the muscles under the arms, *latissimus dorsi*, and the chest muscles). Lean into the wall so that the body's weight is felt on the shoulders, and the upper back bends backwards. Rest with the body's weight on the arms and breathe in and out deeply five times or so.

If you feel an uncomfortable compression in the lower back, move your feet slightly closer to the wall, and try again. It is necessary to be able to relax the muscles on the front of the upper body, so you need to be relatively comfortable in the position.

You may use a partner in this version too, in two ways. The first is to use a small amount of your partner's weight to increase the standard stretch. Placement of the partner's weight is determined by the shape of your back. In general, the partner should place his or her weight on that part of the middle/upper back that is the *least* flexible (that is, most rounded forwards). Have your partner use the flat of the forearm or the hands as shown to transfer the required weight, applying just enough weight to make the exercise strong enough for you. Using a partner tends to concentrate the effect at the point where the weight is applied, and permits you to relax fully in the position. Hold the final position for five breaths or so.

The C–R standing version, a very strong exercise indeed, uses the partner's weight as resistance against which to contract. Here, without letting them slide, try to pull the hands down the wall. This action will contract the muscles mentioned above. Hold for six seconds or so, and cautiously and slowly let yourself relax into the full stretch, ensuring that the arms are pressed completely straight. You must ask your partner to apply his or her weight very sensitively, as this is an extended position where the leverage factors strongly favour the partner.

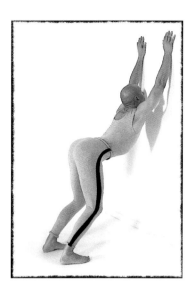

Experiment with different hand spacings too, to find the one most comfortable for the shoulders. Generally, the closer the hands, the stronger the stretch.

All versions are backwards-bending movements, and as such are likely to tighten muscles in the upper or lower back. Back muscles tend to tighten if work is demanded of them towards the contracted end of their range of movement, and most people find it difficult to keep these muscles relaxed while doing movements of this kind. Accordingly, you will feel most comfortable if you follow these exercises with a forwards-bending movement. If the lower back tightens, use exercise 1, or the recovery position of exercise 23 (photograph 5, p. 79). If the upper back has tightened, you may try exercise 8, 11, or exercise 35 overleaf.

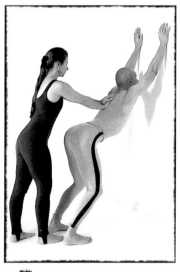

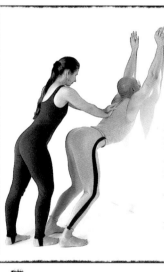

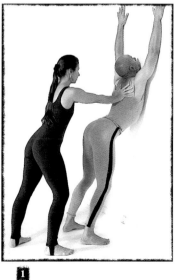

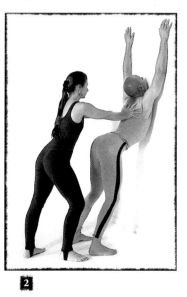

Try different spacing of feet from wall to find most comfortable position

35. *Modified* plough *pose; vertebral isolation*

The *plough* pose of yoga, when performed strictly, requires that the back (from the upper thoracic vertebrae to the lower lumbar vertebrae) be held straight, the body flexed at the hips, and the legs held straight also. Although a beautiful pose to behold, this form necessitates a straight neck to be bent sharply forward at the C7 (lowest cervical vertebra) level. Some physiotherapists and chiropractors believe this to be responsible for some kinds of neck problems. However, a modified plough pose can be a most effective upper back stretch that is safe and relaxing.

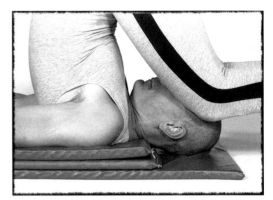

Mats under shoulders reduce neck angle

If performed traditionally, part of the effort felt in the muscles at the back of the neck is due to the legs being held straight. Through hamstring tension and leverage factors, considerable weight can be imposed on the back of the neck. For this reason, at least in the initial stages of working with the pose, the legs should be kept well bent at the knees. In addition, because we wish to use this pose to stretch the upper back, we make no effort to straighten the back, in contrast to the traditional way of doing the pose. If you suspect that your neck is not flexible bending forward, use a folded blanket or similar object *under the back and shoulders only* to reduce the angle the neck will make with the body in the completed position. Having a blanket in this position will not diminish the pose's efficacy as an upper back stretching movement. See the first photograph for details of placement.

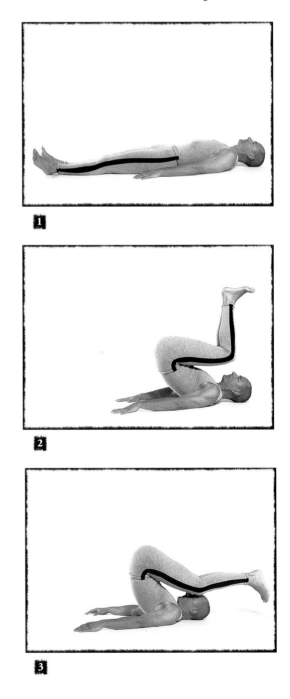

Consider the photographs. Before trying the pose, if you suspect that you may not be able to complete the movement comfortably, place a chair or couch *behind* you, where you expect the legs to come to rest. When you try the position, your legs will rest on the chair, and the difficulty of the pose will be reduced accordingly.

Begin by lying face-up on the floor. If you are thin, you may wish to lie on something comfortable, because the posterior processes of the spine (the visible bumps of the backbone) will contact the floor as you get into and come out of the pose and this may cause discomfort. With an exhalation, lift and bend the legs and, continuing the momentum of this movement, press your hands down to the floor to lift the hips and bring the knees close to the chest. Continue this movement backward. This will lift

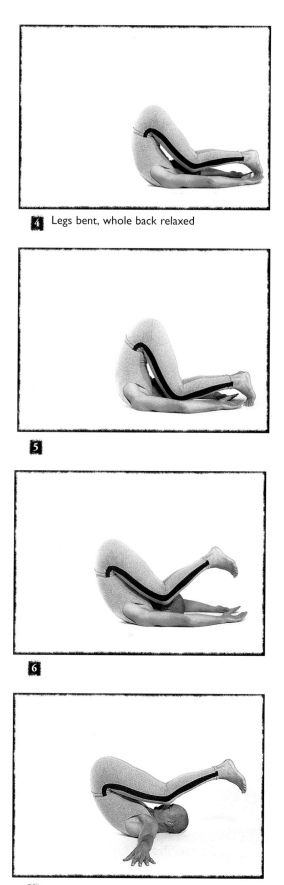

4 Legs bent, whole back relaxed

5

6

7

the body up onto the shoulders and flex the neck forward. Be cautious and do not exceed your capacity to bend at the neck. If you have placed a chair behind you (near your head), rest the legs on it. Otherwise, lower the legs slowly to the floor, keeping the knees flexed. Move your hands behind your head so that you can control precisely the degree of stretch in the neck, as shown. Rest in this position for a few breaths.

To increase the stretch, use the feet to walk the legs very slowly further away behind you. As you do, let the upper back relax completely. Walking the legs away will increase the stretch in both the neck itself (the muscles at the back) and the upper back. Hold the final position for ten breaths or so.

If you wish, you may add a gentle lateral flexion component. Bend both arms at the elbows and hold your waist, and gently incline the body to one side until you feel a stretch in the opposite side of the neck. The body's weight will come onto the hand on the side you are leaning towards. Hold for a breath or two, return to the centre, and try the other side.

To return to the starting position, use the muscles of the lower back, and the arms and shoulders (by pressing back against the floor), to lift the bent legs off the floor, and let the hips fall away from the previous position. As soon as you feel the upper back on the floor, or as soon as you feel your weight moving over the balanced position, take your hands from your waist (or behind you) and place them out to the sides or alongside the body. Use the hands to lower the body slowly to the floor. When the lower back has reached the floor pause for a moment. Rest by letting the legs go down to the floor too.

As mentioned above, whenever we have done a strong stretching movement in one direction it feels good to perform a brief movement in the opposite direction. Accordingly, sit on the floor (or on a chair), straighten the back and open the mouth wide. Slowly incline the head backwards as far as it will go. To complete the stretch, gently close the mouth and clench the teeth. This moves the stretch to the muscles at the front of the neck. Hold for a breath or two and return to the neutral position. Lift the shoulders up and down a few times, and turn the head from side to side.

36. *External hip rotator (piriformis)*

We have found this stretch to be greatly beneficial for some kinds of sciatica, especially if the sciatica is combined with hip pain, and if it has not responded to the previously described hip and hamstring movements. The movement requires some suppleness to get into the starting position, so you may wish to warm up with exercises 7, 9 and 21. An explanation for this muscle's involvement in sciatica and back pain will be found at the end of chapter four.

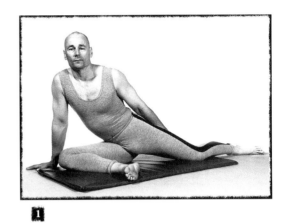

1

The exercise is described for the hip of the right leg. Sit as shown. Your upper body's weight will be supported by your right hand. The objective of the movement is to roll the front of the left leg forwards while keeping the right hip on the floor, with the thighs parallel as seen from above. The effect of this movement is to provide a strong stretch deep inside the right hip. When trying the exercise for the first time, choose a modest knee angle for the front leg to avoid any twisting forces on the knee. If you feel discomfort in the knee, bring the front leg's foot closer to the body. Keep the trunk vertical as you get into the first position.

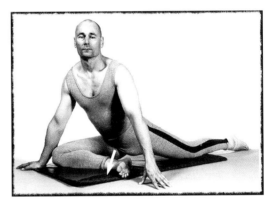

2 C–R: press outside of foot into floor

A C–R stretch can be used to improve the first position. Gently press the outside of the front foot into the floor for six seconds or so. This action contracts *piriformis*. Stop pressing, take a breath in, and on a breath out roll the left leg's hip further across and down to the floor.

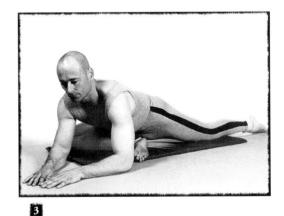

3

The second position requires the upper body to be bent forwards from the hip. Holding the back straight, bend forwards from the hips, inclining the centre of the body towards the ankle of the front foot, rather that towards the knee, the more comfortable direction. So doing will provide a powerful stretch for *piriformis* (one of the external hip rotators) in the right hip, in addition to the muscles inside the front leg, the adductors.

The C–R stretch may be performed again, from the second position. Hold for five breaths and repeat for the other side. Compare left and right. To make the stretch more effective as you become more flexible, open out the angle of the lower leg with respect to the knee, keeping the front thigh as close to parallel with the back leg as possible.

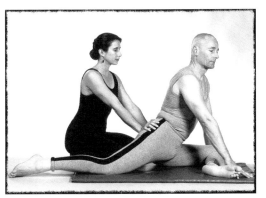

1 Partner rolls hip of back leg across and forwards to the floor

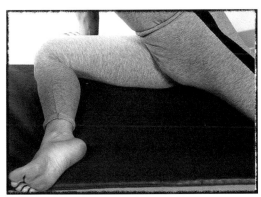

2

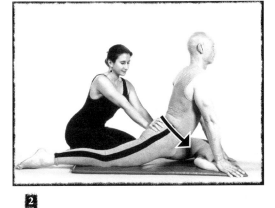

Easiest stretch position: flexed knee

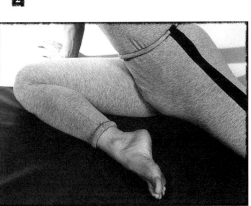

Most difficult stretch position: knee 90 degrees

A partner can help in this movement too, by holding the hip of the front leg on the floor, while leaning weight across and down on the hip of the back leg. So doing will reduce the effort needed to hold yourself in the stretch position. The C–R stretch is more easily performed with a partner for the same reason.

This completes the stretching exercises. For notes about the best frequency of stretching workouts, see the final section of chapter one. For combinations of exercises for problem areas, see p. 182. We shall now go to chapter three, which discusses how to strengthen the body to provide a measure of prevention for the future.

STRENGTHENING EXERCISES

This chapter considers the standard ways of thinking about strengthening exercises from which our approach will be drawn. As noted in the previous chapters, knowing *why* one is doing something a certain way is just as important as knowing how. Thus this chapter provides a brief outline of the development of each of the approaches to strengthening exercise in addition to the more technical aspects of the approach I advocate .

Isometric

The term isometric refers to a technique of developing strength using a strong contraction of the muscles without any change in the *length* of the muscles used during the exercise (hence the technical term '*static* contraction'). Isometric exercise regimens have been the subject of a large number of experiments that have demonstrated they are effective. Isometric exercises are contractions made against immovable objects, where you push or pull against the resistance as hard as you can for six to ten seconds. For example, if you press your palms together in front of your chest you will feel the chest, front shoulder, and the muscles of the back of your arm (*triceps*) contract. This is the standard isometric exercise for these muscles. Another example is to stand in a doorway, with the backs of your hands against the frame. An effective isometric contraction for the lateral shoulder muscles is to press the backs of the hands against the frame (out to the sides) for between six to ten seconds while holding the arms straight.

Although few researchers doubt the effectiveness of this approach, questions remain about the extent of the strength gains with respect to the associated joint's whole range of movement. Some researchers have claimed that the strength gains reported are specific to the position of the limb when used to perform the exercise. This is significant because, in the normal way of doing isometric exercises, muscular effort is expended only in one particular part of the range. It is possible to do isometric exercise at different points in the range, but the design of the body frequently lends itself to useful and convenient isometric exercise only in certain positions. For example, with respect to the chest/shoulder exercise mentioned, critics claim that these muscles become strong only in the position the hands and arms are held while performing the contractions. However, there is nothing in the method itself to prevent the user from employing an almost infinite number of variations of the contraction position.

Another reservation is that isometric exercises require greater motivation than other systems. It is claimed that persons using these systems become stale more quickly than with other approaches. Although there may be some truth in this claim, it is due more to the fact that strength gains are a matter of perception with isometrics; that is, there is no easy way to see strength gains while using the system in the same way as when you use weights. This is probably a genuine shortcoming of isometrics, as one of the undoubted benefits of conventional weight training is the visual proof of strength increases every time you add even a small weight to the bar—immediate positive feedback, in other words. However, there is nothing to prevent persons training with isometrics from testing themselves with other conventional strength measuring techniques from time to time.

These reservations are of little concern to us here. With few exceptions (noted below), we shall mainly use isometrics for stretching. In the C–R approach to stretching, the isometric contractions are always made at the **end** of the useable range of movement, and mainly to increase flexibility—any increase in strength resulting from its application is a bonus. An increase in flexibility *per se* is neither a good nor a bad thing—it depends entirely on the context. For example, ballet dancers are the only athletes who routinely suffer stress fractures of the hip. Their extreme flexibility, acquired over many years of hard training, means that the joint can be stressed in ways for which it is not ideally structured. More specifically, in a dance movement performed at or near the end of the range of movement, the joint itself takes more of the forces generated than is usually the case. These considerations are not of concern to us, except for the general lesson that it is preferable to develop strength and flexibility together. Using the C–R method guarantees that we are not only developing flexibility, we are also developing additional strength precisely in the areas needed.

Isotonic

Isotonic exercise refers to techniques to acquire strength which use muscle contractions against a resistance that can move. Such forces may be generated to push or pull a weight or some other resistance (*concentric* contractions), or to resist the movement of some object (as in lowering something heavy to the floor, called *eccentric* contractions). Both approaches are effective in building strength. This approach to strength training is not new. Milos of Croton, a famous wrestler of ancient Greece, was said to have lifted a bull calf overhead every day until it was fully grown. We do not necessarily need extensive gym equipment to do isotonic training. The body itself can be effective resistance, as in doing chin-ups or similar exercises. We shall be using the weight of the body in some of the resistance exercises described below.

There is no doubt that isotonic training is successful in achieving its goals, and this approach to strength training is the method of choice of the overwhelming majority of athletes who need strength for their sports. Nonetheless, even though there is positive visual and physical feedback, this kind of training still requires motivation. One needs to persevere with strength training for more than two months, which seems to be a threshold for many people. Beyond this period the drop-out rate from the strength classes I teach is very small.

Matching training to expected demand

There seems to be a threshold effect in most people—no exercise or too much. The intention of this section is to mention a few common-sense suggestions upon which to base a training schedule to suit you. The main reasons exercise regimens fail is because there is no clearly visualised goal (purpose) to the program, or because the exercise program is inappropriate. Let us consider these reasons in turn.

Without a goal, any exercise program is likely to become perfunctory at best, or mechanical and unfeeling at worst. Either disposition means little incentive to continue, and increased risk of injury. Too often, people with the best and apparently the strongest of intentions cease their routines after a week or two. Those of you who have had a neck or back problem are usually more motivated to continue, at least while the exercises seem to be alleviating the problem. Unfortunately, ending the program when you get better is leaving the job half done. Your 'pre-injury state of fitness' was precisely the set of physical characteristics that contributed to the problem in the first place. It is necessary to strengthen the body against the likelihood of a recurrence. If this is your goal, you do not need a comprehensive gym training program, but you do need a number of specific strengthening exercises of the sort that can be done at home. The critical point is that you do need to *do* them.

If you are a weekend athlete, such as a golf or tennis player, and you have a history of back or neck problems, you will need a few additional exercises. Such activities, with their demands on spinal extension with rotation, require strong waist and back muscles. The asymmetrical nature of these kinds of sports compounds the problem. However, if sufficient strength is developed, such activities can be pursued safely. The more effective (higher intensity) exercises will be required, and although the exercises are shown in a gymnasium setting, a little ingenuity will allow you to perform them at home.

Low back pain is particularly common among athletes. Certain sports are especially prone to this problem (sweep rowing, for example) due to the asymmetrical nature of the activity. Other athletes merely require strong waist muscles to transfer power or strength from one half of the body to the other. Athletes should explore the whole range of strengthening exercises presented.

Details of numbers of repetitions of exercises and frequency of training are set out in the *Planning a total routine section* at the end of this chapter.

POST-REHABILITATION
STRENGTHENING EXERCISES

37. Modified dynamic yoga rotations (lying)

This movement and its variants are perhaps the most important strengthening exercises for the lower back. Although included in the strengthening section, it is both a strengthening and a stretching exercise when performed to the extent of your range of movement. Additionally, if the source of your back pain is the *quadratus lumborum* (refer to exercise 17, *legs apart* near the beginning of chapter two), this exercise done in its easiest form can ease the pain of an attack considerably.

No matter what your overall level of strength, you must begin the exercise in the minimum resistance configuration (legs completely bent at the knees). Look at the photographs. Notice that the hands are palm down, pressing on the floor. This stabilises the shoulders, and holds them onto the floor. If your legs are relatively heavy, you will need to press quite hard to keep the shoulders on the floor. At this stage, the thighs are vertical, and the heels held near the bottom.

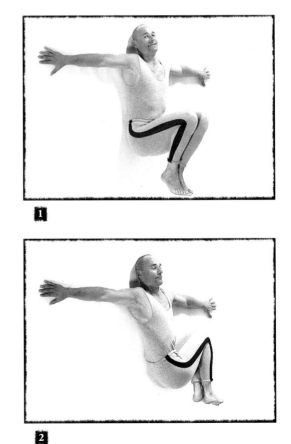

Let your legs and hips roll to one side, aiming the knees at one hand. This instruction is vital to avoid hyperextending the spine, and essential to achieving the stretch in the lower back. Once you feel the weight of the legs (in the muscles of the waist and lower back), gently lower the legs as close to the floor as you can, keeping the knees aimed at the hand on that side. Try not to rest the legs on the floor. This is the stretch phase. Rest a few breaths in and out in the final position. Then, with an exhalation, *slowly* lift the legs back up to the starting position by using the muscles of the waist. Of course, the muscles of the arms and shoulders will be working too, in a support role, but try as much as possible to use the muscles of the waist to lift the legs. This is the strengthening part. Repeat the movement several times with the legs in the completely bent position, from one side to the other.

If you are able to do this with no discomfort, and are able to hold the shoulders against the floor, you may increase both the stretch and the resistance by partially

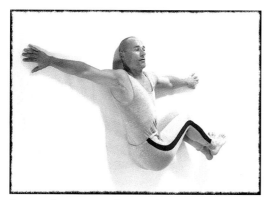

Intermediate version (legs partly extended)

Correct form in exercise 37

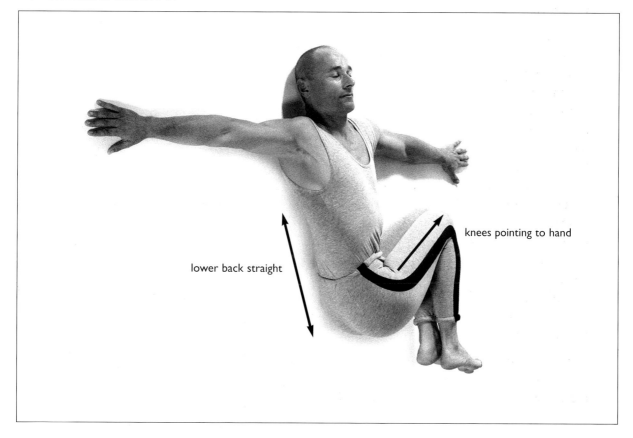

lower back straight

knees pointing to hand

straightening the legs. Try to hold the knees together while doing the movement, but maintain the angle; that is, check that regardless of the position of the lower leg, the thighs are pointing at your hand.

The strongest stretch (and consequently the strongest resistance in the strengthening phase) is when you can hold the legs straight throughout the movement. *This is an advanced movement* and you must work up to it slowly. Building up to the exercise at this level of difficulty could take many months. Do not sacrifice form to do the exercise with straight legs.

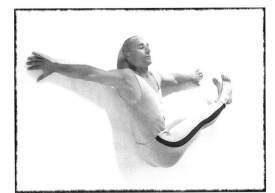

Advanced version (legs straight)

Pay attention to whether lowering and lifting the legs on one side is more difficult than the other. This is usually the case. The side that feels the weaker or less flexible (that is, does not go as close to the floor), must determine how many repetitions are done for the other side. You need to find out which side has the lesser capacity (of either strength or flexibility) and do only that number of repetitions for the other side too. This will ensure that the weaker or tighter side will catch up with the other because it is experiencing the greater stimulus for change.

Alternatively, when you know which side is the weaker or tighter, you may change the approach to the movement by doing the exercise from the starting position (legs vertical) and only lowering and raising the legs to the one side. When you can do no more, rest for a moment and repeat for the other side, doing only the same number. For strengthening, it is preferable to work one side at a time because the muscles have far less time to rest between contractions.

Do not do too many of these movements initially. This is a very strong exercise, and you will need to work up to it slowly. As with the stretching movements, err on the side of doing too little in the beginning. For women, developing the requisite arm and shoulder strength may be the limiting factor in the first instance.

Breathing in a particular way can help you in this exercise. Breathe in while the legs are vertical, and hold the breath as you lower the legs. Breathe out as you lift the legs. When holding the breath, do not take in a deeper breath than normal. By not breathing out during the lowering phase you will achieve two things: the trunk the trunk is made stronger by the *Valsalva manoeuvre* (the compression of the abdominal contents by the muscles of the trunk); and the exhalation makes you a little stronger in the exertion phase. Do not exaggerate these suggestions.

38. *Abdominal curls (floor/chair) or* crunches

This is the basic abdominal strength exercise. Some years ago, researchers in the United States realised that the conventional sit-up exercise (wherein one's feet were held under a support with either straight or bent knees and the body lifted up until the face contacted the knees) was potentially very harmful to the lower back. However, whenever you visit a gym, you will see this movement being done. You should appreciate why this exercise is both bad for the back and an inefficient abdominal strengthening exercise.

Any sitting-up movement (used as a strength exercise) where the lower back is lifted from the floor places a strain on the lower back. The hip flexors play a role as shapers of the lumbar lordosis, and in the inability of some people to lie face-up with the lower back on the floor (see exercise 7, *modified* salute to the sun). Anatomically (*psoas* and *iliacus* will be considered as one muscle for simplicity), the hip flexors originate in the transverse processes of the lumbar spine and insert at the top of the femur. This means that when they contract strongly against fixed legs (as in the conventional sit-up) the body's weight is lifted from the front of the lower back. This is a class II lever, with the effort between fulcrum and load, as shown in the illustration. The main significance of this class of lever, with respect to the arrangement of the bones of the spine, is the generation in the lumbar vertebrae of powerful shear forces, which can disturb their ideal position. Additionally, if the abdominal muscles are weak (the usual reason for doing the exercise) the upper body is apt to lag slightly behind the waist as the body is lifted, and this hyperextends the spine while compressing it. Compression forces alone can irritate the facet joints, whose articular surfaces are rich in nerves. In most people the hip flexors are far stronger than the abdominal muscles. If stabilising the pelvis in the horizontal plane is one of our goals, this strength imbalance needs to be addressed. The conventional sit-up will only increase the imbalance, as its major effect is to strengthen the hip flexors. It is only when the abdominal muscles are really strong that this exercise can be done without the lower back taking the strain. In any case, this exercise should be avoided by anyone with back problems.

Why the conventional situp can injure the lower back

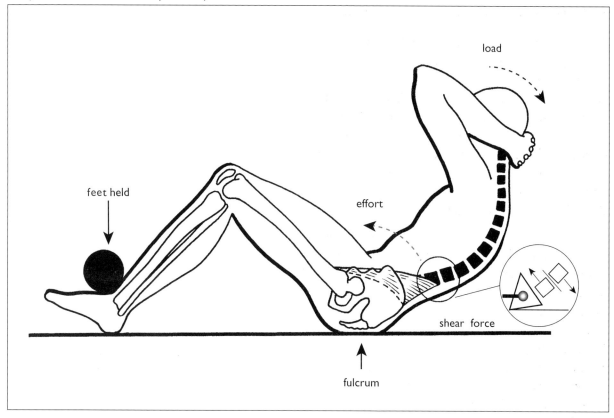

feet held

load

effort

shear force

fulcrum

Class II lever

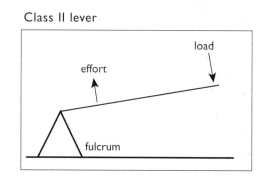

effort

load

fulcrum

Consider the anatomy of the abdominal muscles for a moment (for simplicity only the *rectus abdominus* will be mentioned). Their origin is the cartilages of the lower ribs; their insertion is the pubic bone. Their only action therefore is to bring the ribs closer to the pubic bone (or the pubic bone closer to the ribs if the ribs are fixed)—they have no direct role in hip flexion at all. To be effective as a strengthener of the abdominal muscles, the sit-up exercise needs to be redesigned. In the conventional sit-up, the only part of the movement that can strengthen these muscles is actually avoided. If the movement is done quickly (as it usually is when people are trying to do as many as possible), the action of lifting the head off the floor rapidly is initiated by the neck, arm and back muscles. This momentum is used to help the abdominal muscles contract as the shoulders are lifted from the floor, and the hip flexors take over completing the movement.

The only way to make this an *abdominal* exercise is to isolate the abdominal muscles. This is done by flexing the hips as shown (the lower legs may be rested on a chair for greater comfort), and doing the exercise *slowly*. Place just the fingertips on the temples (this stops you lifting the head with your arms), and slowly lift the head up with the muscles of the neck until the chin comes close to the chest. Focusing the effort in the abdominal muscles, curl the shoulders off the floor towards the hips while breathing out. Do not let the lower back come off the floor. If the exercise is done properly, you will notice the lower back being pressed onto the floor even harder. This shows the role of the abdominal muscles in flattening the lumbar curve. Once you have curled up as far as you can, hold the final position for a second or two, lower yourself back to the floor, and breathe in. If you find that the body's weight is too great, fold your hands across your chest and try again. If this is still too difficult, hold your hands by your sides. Work up to doing ten repetitions. Remember to do the exercise sufficiently slowly so that each increment of movement is produced by a contraction of the relevant muscle—never use momentum to lift yourself up.

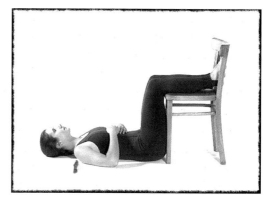

1

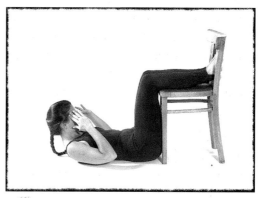

2

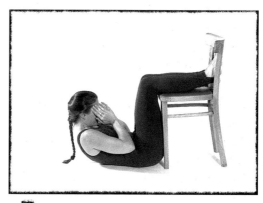

3

39. Back uncurls (over flat or curved bench)

The conventional strengthening exercise for the back muscles involves lying face-down, and with the arms in a suitable position (determined by one's strength). The head and shoulders are lifted from the floor by arching the back, and in some versions the legs are also lifted. One problem with this exercise is that the muscles are expected to work outside their normal range of movement.

The demands of normal daily life are to straighten a *bent* back. In the exercise just described, the muscles are required to *hyperextend* an already straight spine further backwards to an arched position. The risk of irritating structures involved in the original back pain is considerable. The pain may be muscular in origin or the result of compression of the joints of the spine. There is a very real risk of the muscles involved becoming cramped by this demand, or going into spasm—just because they are being asked to do work outside their normal range of movement. Any muscle working outside its normal range of movement is likely to cramp, especially if the demand is made in the strongly contracted part of its range. The final problem is one of specificity, a principle of strength training. Muscles respond by becoming stronger in the range of movement trained. Any strength gains made in the hyperextended range using the standard exercise are unlikely to be useful in daily life activities.

The following exercise is designed to avoid these pitfalls. It demands effort from the back muscles in the range of movements required in daily life. The movement requires a padded bench, a firm cylindrical cushion, or the wide padded end of a strong couch. Any surface over which you can drape the body will do, providing it will support you safely. When attempting to strengthen the muscles of a 'problem' back, it is better to have the whole spine supported. In this exercise, the whole spine is supported, and after some practice you will be able to work the back muscles through a wide range of movement.

Always choose a support with a wide radius for your first attempts. If there are no adverse reactions, you can decrease the radius of the support so that the

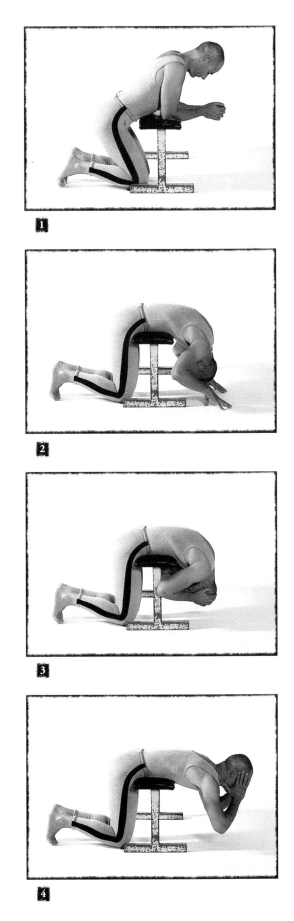

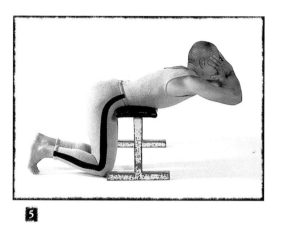

5

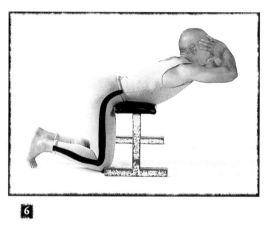

6

strengthening and stretching effects are experienced through a wider range. Remember, the smaller the radius, the greater the range through which the body can bend backwards and the stronger the effects will be.

Look at the photographs. Begin by lying face-down over the support. The hips are flexed and the whole body relaxed. The starting position is similar to the final position of the abdominal strengthening exercise (but upside down). This movement can be considered the reverse of the last exercise.

Place the fingertips against the temples and tuck the chin as close to the chest as you can; this flexes the spine forward. This exercise is called the *back uncurl*, to remind you of how it is to be done—you 'peel' or 'uncurl' the body off the support, beginning with the head. After lifting the head up, breathe in. Contract the muscles of the upper back, then those of the middle of the back, and finally those of the lower back. Do not lift the whole body off the support because this would involve the bottom muscles as well, and would take the body away from the support. Instead, just as you press

Normal and hyperextended positions of spine

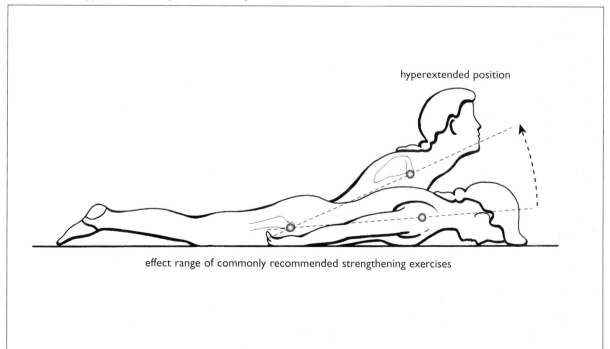

hyperextended position

effect range of commonly recommended strengthening exercises

the lower back into the floor in the abdominal exercise discussed in the previous section, you need to feel the support pressing quite hard into the lower abdominal area to be sure that the spine remains supported. You do not need to arch much above the point when the back is straight. Breathe out as you lower yourself to the starting position. Note that breathing is not easy in this exercise because of the weight of the body on the abdominal area.

The first sequence of photographs shows the exercise over a flat bench. The second sequence shows it over a purpose-built support. The barrels are 50 litre drums cut lengthwise, with four legs and internal bracing. They can also be made from 200 litre drums, for larger or less flexible people. You may be able to make something similar, or ask a welding shop to do the job. This 'low-tech' approach gives excellent results for both stretching and strengthening exercises.

Start by trying to do the movement as described. In the beginning, many people try to do the movement by lifting the whole body off the support, but this will not do. You need to *uncurl*; that is, the back muscles need to be contracted individually, from the uppermost (the neck muscles) all the way down to the lowest. Notice that although the neck muscles experience only the weight of the head, the resistance being applied to the muscles of the back *increases* as more of the body is lifted. This matches the demands of daily life almost perfectly. Once you can do ten slow repetitions, you can use a small weight behind the neck—even a book will do. Breathe out as you return to the starting position, and breathe in as soon as you lift the head. Ensure that you do the movement slowly so that momentum does not help you. As with the abdominal exercise, every increment of movement must be the result of a greater force having been applied. If you have trouble emulating the movement as described, you may wish to refer to the photographs and descriptions of exercise 45, *Hyperextension,* below. A comparison will make the differences clear.

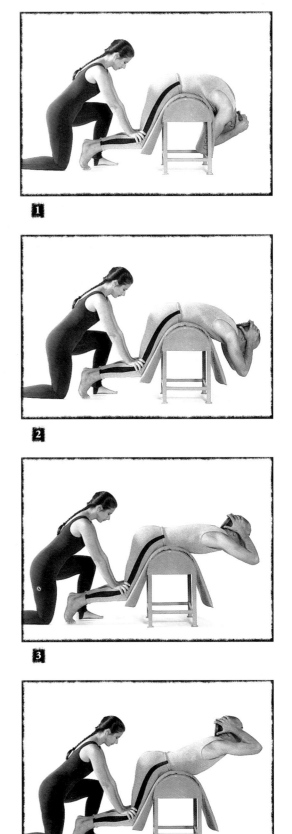

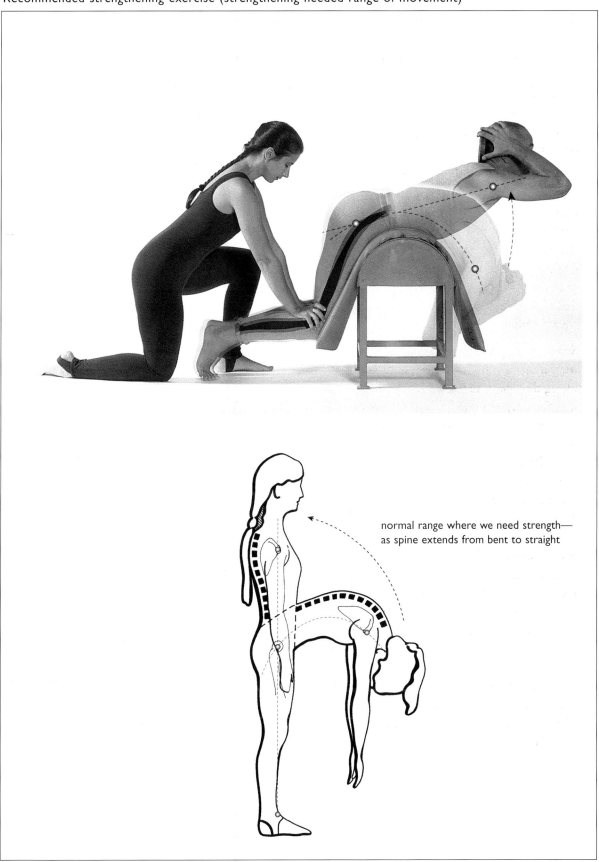

normal range where we need strength—
as spine extends from bent to straight

127

40. Neck curls

Recall the position we used to give the neck a gentle stretch backwards. From this position we can strengthen the front neck muscles, which often are relatively weak. Lower the head into the stretched position as detailed in chapter one (exercise 12, *Neck extension over support*). Now, instead of lifting the head with the hands as before, use the muscles at the front of the throat to bring the head back to horizontal, all the while bringing the chin towards the chest. Help these muscles with your hands if necessary. For the first few weeks of doing this exercise, do not let the head go backwards to anywhere near what you consider the limits of this movement; wait until the front neck muscles are strong enough to return the head easily before letting the head go further back. Because you are working from the edge of the mattress, the further the head goes back the better it is supported, if your body is in the suggested position. We are aiming for ten, slow repetitions of this movement before we consider the neck to be sufficiently strong for daily life. If you require more strength for a particular purpose, you may attempt the movement unsupported, after having achieved the ten repetitions in the manner described. Breathe in while stretching backwards, and out as you lift the head.

Ensure that the whole neck is bending backwards. This means that not only is the head as a whole moving backwards, but the chin is also moving backwards *with respect to the neck* during the movement. In the second sequence of photographs I am holding a credit card between my teeth to illustrate the two components of this complex movement. Do not go too far backwards— only as far back as you can control with the neck muscles.

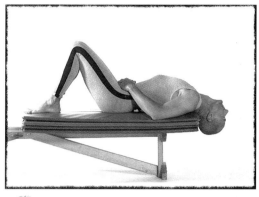

1

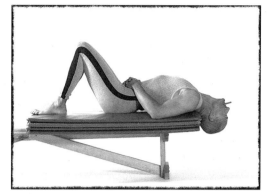

1

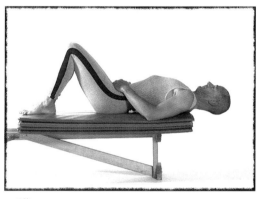

2

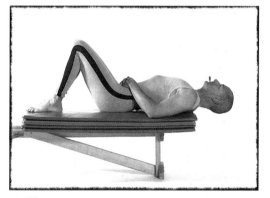

2

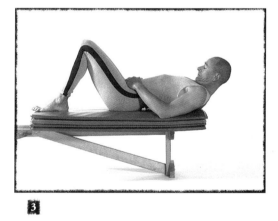

3

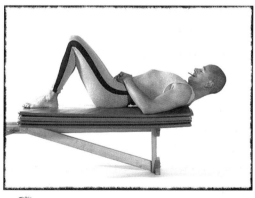

3

ADVANCED STRENGTHENING EXERCISES (PREVENTION)

41. Hanging knee lifts

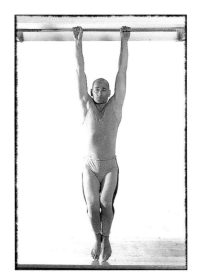

This is the premier abdominal muscle strengthening exercise. It is also the most difficult. You must not attempt this unless you can do ten or more slow repetitions of the abdominal curls described above, in exercise 38. It is best to do this exercise with a partner, as it lends itself to being done 'negatively'. If this exercise is too difficult, an easier version is described at the end of this section.

Thus far we have been using concentric strength building movements; that is, we have been contracting the muscles we are trying to strengthen against a resistance. Eccentric strength exercises have the muscles do work by *lowering* a weight. In this form of training, you demand work of the muscles by making them resist elongation by a force or weight. Such repetitions are usually called 'negatives'. Any weight training exercise can be done in this way, but there are a few disadvantages. One is that you need a partner to help you do the work during the concentric phase (the partner lifts the weight or the body to a starting position from which you will lower it). Another is the fact that in eccentric movements you are about 40% stronger than in concentric ones. This means that you will need to be handling significantly heavier weights than you would normally, with consequently greater risk of injury and greater muscle soreness following training. Some researchers claim this increased soreness is because the tendons (where they join the muscles) take more of the strain than they do in concentric training. Nonetheless, some exercises lend themselves very well to negative training, and the *hanging knee lift* is a perfect example.

It is worth mentioning at this point that although negative training is not so often used in the weight training gym, it is the most commonly used method for teaching strength moves in gymnastics. Negative training simply involves lowering a weight that is too heavy to lift normally, in a *slow and controlled* way. The negative phase of the movement should take three to five seconds, depending on momentum considerations and the range of movement involved—the greater the range the more time it should take.

Back to the exercise. The movement requires lifting the knees as closely as possible to the chest. Many of you may recognise the movement from the gym, but this version has been modified in

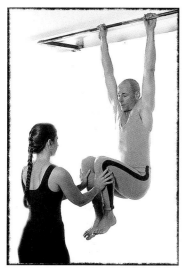

Start position

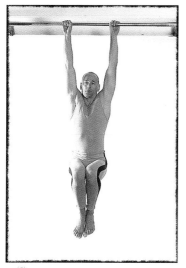

1

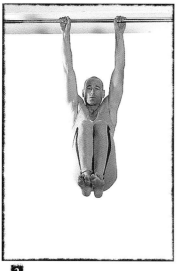

2

significant ways. In the conventional form, you hang from a bar or from an elbow support with the legs hanging down. The legs are then swung up; one version letting the knees bend, and the other keeping the legs straight. The problem with both these versions is similar to problems with the conventional sit-up—the powerful hip flexors move the legs in the first 90 degrees (or more) of the knee lift and the resulting momentum completes the movement. To see why this is significant, stand on one leg with one hand feeling the abdominal muscles. Lift one knee up to about horizontal, and you will find that the stomach muscles in fact do not contract at all. Even when the knees are lifted together, the hip flexors do most of the work in the first 90 degrees of movement. This means the exercise, as it is normally done, will not strengthen the muscles it is supposed to.

The way to overcome the use of the hip flexors is as follows. Grasp the bar firmly and hang from it. Ask your partner to hold your legs below the knees, and lift the knees up until they are horizontal. Have your partner take away his or her hands. *Slowly* lift the knees as high as you can towards the chest. Even if you can only lift the knees a fraction of an inch, persevere with the exercise. In this case, you are doing a mostly isometric contraction, and simply holding the knees in this position makes the abdominal muscles stronger if you try hard. This is the first phase.

Let us assume that you were able to do two repetitions, and struggled to do a couple more, without actually being able to lift the knees. Now we use the negative approach. Ask your partner to lift the knees as close to the chest as possible, and you try to hold them there. Hold the position for a second if you can, and then slowly lower the knees to the horizontal starting position. Immediately, have your partner lift the knees back to the chest. Again, you hold and then slowly lower them. As the muscles become more fatigued, your capacity to lower your legs slowly decreases, and the legs fall to the starting position more and more quickly. As soon as you cannot control the lowering (and the knees drop as soon as your partner lets them go), stop. Try only a few of these 'negatives' the first time you attempt the exercise— if you do too many of them your stomach muscles will be sore for *days*. Make haste slowly. If you are not able to do negatives with the full weight of the legs, have your partner take some of the weight and try hard to control the remainder.

Always breathe out strongly as you lift the knees (a full breath will hinder the completion of the movement) and breathe in as you lower the legs. Because this exercise is strenuous, you may find that you need extra breaths in and out, especially if you are working negatively. Breathe where it feels most natural.

One of the reasons this movement is so successful is that it stretches the whole upper body in the starting position. When you lift the knees to the chest in this exercise, many muscles are involved besides the complex of abdominal muscles. The muscles in between the ribs (*intercostals*), the back muscles under the arms, and the arm muscles themselves are all at work, just trying to hang onto the bar.

When you feel confident with the movement, ask your partner to stand to one side and watch you do it. If you are doing it correctly, the normal lumbar curve should flatten, then round out as you complete the exercise. The abdominal muscles span the ribs and the pubic bones, so that if they are contracting the shape of the lumbar curve must change. It is possible for someone with good hip flexibility to lift the knees very close to the chest using only the hip flexors. This will not work the abdominal muscles as much as we want. Such people should do the negative version, and the partner must lift the knees high enough that the lumbar spine curves forward. This may require the knees to be taken past the armpits.

An easier version of this exercise requires an adjustable incline board. I have shown this movement on an incline board that uses a set of 'ladder bars' for its support. Look at the photographs on the page overleaf.

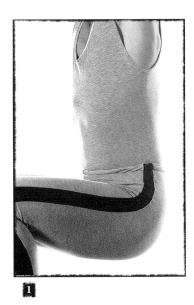

1

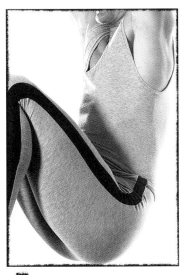

2

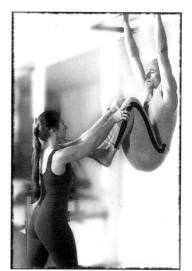

Doing negatives

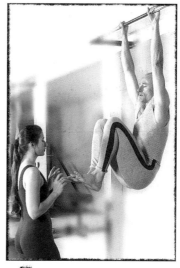

1

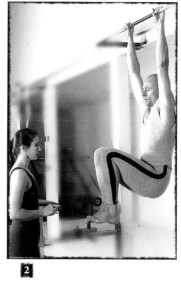

2

I am holding the ladder bars with a supinated (palms facing shoulders) grip, as the arm muscles are in their strongest positions this way. If you do not have access to ladder bars, hold the edges of the incline board itself above your head to stabilise the upper body. Without lifting the body, slowly lift the legs with the knees bent as close to your chest as you can. You will reach a point where any further movement of the knees towards the chest will lift the hips off the board. This indicates the starting position. Note that a combination of hip flexibility and muscle attachments will result in different starting positions for everybody. Typically, women's starting positions will have the knees closer to their chests than men's. Some people can bring their knees all the way back to their chests. If this is the case, you will need to have the knees far enough apart so that when you do the exercise you can take the knees *past* the body, under the arms.

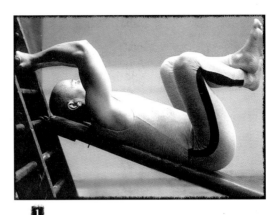

From the starting position, the exercise is done as described above, by *slowly* lifting the knees towards (or past) the chest until the abdominal muscles are fully contracted. Be careful that you are not merely lifting the whole body off the board with the strength of the arm and back muscles. As with the hanging knee lift, each increment of contraction of the abdominal muscles must produce a change in the shape of the spine, from straight in the starting position to the curved contracted position. To be sure, have your partner check your form. Stop lifting when the upper back begins to lift off the board. Do not use a sudden movement of the knees to generate momentum to achieve the movement. Slower is better here—as you will quickly feel. Adjust the incline to a steeper angle as you become stronger.

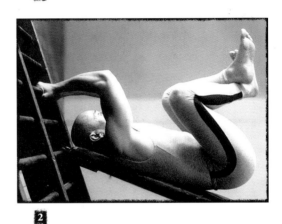

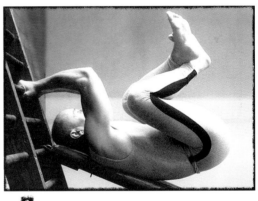

Your partner may help in the following ways. For the first month or two, ask your partner to assist you to complete a few additional repetitions after you no longer can complete repetitions by yourself. When you feel ready, you can extend this 'failure zone' by asking your partner to add negatives after you have completed the assisted positives described. Have your partner lift the knees to or past the chest; immediately your partner lets the knees go, try to hold them there. After a second or so, take four to five seconds to lower the legs to the starting position. Repeat this for a few additional repetitions.

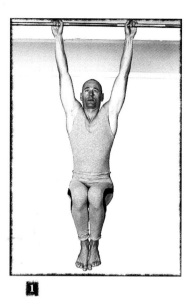

1

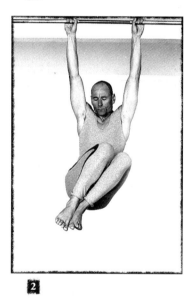

2

42. Hanging knee lifts with lateral flexion

In this version of the exercise, lift one hip higher than the other as you lift the knees up to the chest. This will affect the side waist muscles (*obliques*) as well as the abdominals, and the muscles in between the ribs (*intercostals*) on the side you are lifting towards. This movement must be done slowly to be effective; that is, take a few seconds at least to complete one repetition—first to one side then to the other. To reduce the strain of hanging from the bar for too long, you can do the repetitions for one side, get down off the bar and rest, and do the repetitions for the other side a little later. To make sure the waist muscles develop evenly over time if you follow this approach, begin with the left side on one training day, and on the next training day begin with the right side. Breathing is the same as the previous exercise.

43. Abdominal curls (over support)

The barrel shown in the photographs is discussed above, in exercise 39, p. 126. The curved surface ensures that the contraction of the abdominal muscles is progressive, and through a much wider range of movement than in the floor abdominal exercise detailed above. An additional benefit of working on a curved surface is that we can smoothly change the angle through which we want the muscles to work, and the part of the spine in contact with the surface of the barrel is supported. Although you may not have such objects lying around the house, a little ingenuity will locate a substitute. Whatever you used to do the back uncurl above will also work well for this exercise. Try to work up to doing ten slow repetitions. As with the abdominal curl, breathe in as you stretch backwards, and out as you curl up.

This exercise may be intensified by using a small weight, as with the floor abdominal crunch. If you do use a weight (a book or similar object), do not be surprised if you feel the main effects in the muscles of the front of the neck for the first few weeks.

Look at the photographs. Note the way the body is stretching over the barrel in the first frame. Lower yourself into this position slowly and relax there for a moment to stretch. Make sure that you do this over a curvature which is suitable for you (not too small a radius). A larger support is better than a small one at first.

When you attempt this for the first time, do not allow yourself to go back as far as you think you can. Rather, cautiously let yourself go back part of the way only. Then lift your head towards your chest, and begin lifting your shoulders off the support, trying (as in the abdominal curl) to curl up into as tight a ball as possible. Do not try to lift your lower back from the support, because this will engage the hip flexors. The next time you lower yourself to the starting position, let yourself go down a little further; after a few repetitions let yourself go down as far as you can. In this way the initial repetitions become your warm-up. The need to do the movement slowly cannot be over-emphasised—each increment of forward movement must be by muscle contraction *alone* and not by momentum.

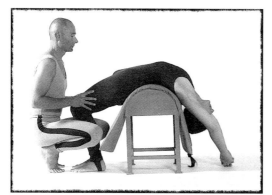

Stretch first

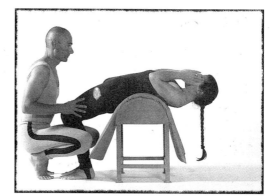

2

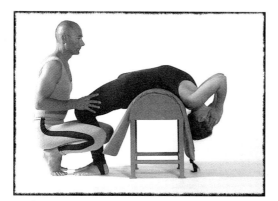

1

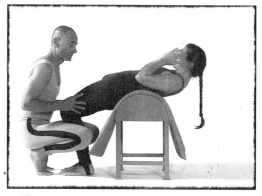

3

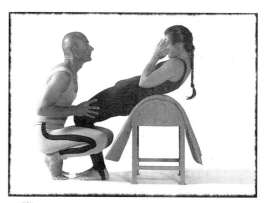

4

44. Lying lateral curls (over support)

As the photographs show, a similar movement may be done for the side waist muscles (*obliques*). Try to position yourself on the support so that you only use the waist muscles to lift yourself. This means that the centre of your body (that is, the soft part of the side of the waist, between the hip and the lowest rib) should be roughly over the highest part of the support. It is possible to lift the body from the support, but with similar reservations as with the abdominal movement described above (that is, if you do lift the waist off the support, you will be using one of the hip muscles (*tensor fascia lata*) and the purpose of the exercise as described here will be defeated). The lifting movement must be similar to the exercise above. Try to bring the side of your waist as close to the hip as possible (a sideways curl of the body) and do not lift the waist itself from the support. Breathe out as you exert the effort, and in as you return to the start position.

Repeat for the other side, and as with all exercises which permit comparison, compare left with right.

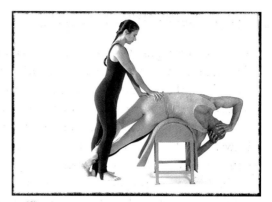

1

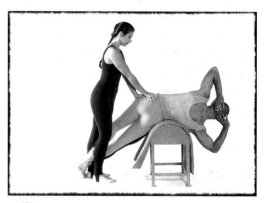

2

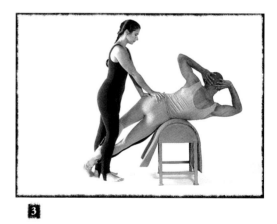

3

45. Hyperextensions

This is a much mis-performed movement in gyms around the world. In the way it is usually done, it is partly a back exercise, and partly a hip extensor and hamstring exercise. In the way described here, the exercise is almost wholly a hip and hamstring exercise, with the back muscles relegated to a support role.

Although the exercise is demonstrated from a hyperextension bench especially designed for the purpose, you can duplicate the movement if you have a partner and a strong table. Place sufficient padding on the surface of the table, with a chair on the floor in front of where you expect to hang. Lie face-down on the table and, using the chair, move yourself off the edge of the table until the hip joints are past the edge. Ask your partner to support you in this position by sitting astride your legs, taking care that your knees are not being pressed too hard into the top of the table. Once securely in position, move the chair out of the way to do the movement. When you finish, bring the chair back again to help you get out of the position.

Let yourself hang from the support as shown with the back held straight. This places the hamstring muscles under mild stretch. The angle your body will make with respect to the support will depend on your hamstring muscles' flexibility. Do not sacrifice straightness of the lower back for an apparent increase in this angle by letting the body hang closer to the floor than the straight-back position will permit.

Have your partner watch the material of your shirt covering your lower back. The exercise is performed properly if the shirt does not wrinkle above the waist, indicating that the lower back muscles have remained the same length throughout the movement. Your pants should wrinkle below your bottom muscles, indicating that both the hip extensors (*gluteus maximus*) and the three hamstring muscles are extending the body with respect to the hip joint. Because a small contraction of these muscles produces a large movement of the head, it is even more important with this movement than some others that you do it slowly. Do not lift yourself above horizontal. For minimum resistance, use body weight only (this is quite sufficient) and with the hands folded

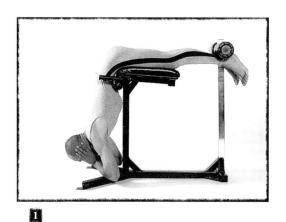

1

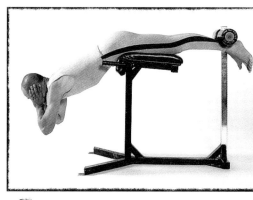

2

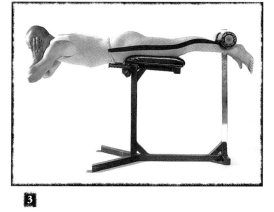

3

over the chest or held at your sides. To increase slightly, place the fingers lightly against the temples. To increase resistance further, use a light weight behind the head (or to remove any potential neck strain, use a heavier one held against the chest). Breathe out as you lift yourself up, and in as you lower yourself to the starting position.

This exercise, together with exercise 39, the *back uncurl*, forms the strengthening components of a common, essential function, that of straightening the back and extending the back with respect to the legs. Breaking this complex movement down into two parts permits safe strengthening of all the back muscles involved. Added to suitable rotation and abdominal strengthening movements, powerful trunk function can be developed.

46. Straight-arm dumbbell rows

This is the second of the exercises presented designed to increase the strength of those muscles involved in rotation of the shoulders with respect to the hips (see also exercise 37). The distinguishing characteristic of this movement is that, in addition to strengthening the waist muscles (internal and external obliques, the front abdominals, and the lower back muscles), it strengthens the muscles involved in *scapular* retraction (pulling of the shoulder rearwards and inwards). For this reason, athletes or others requiring strength in rotation that stresses shoulder involvement (for example, sweep rowers) may find this movement useful.

One other group of people may find this exercise beneficial. Observation suggests that one characteristic of the ageing person is the tendency towards an increased forward curvature of the upper back, called *kyphosis*. In good posture (see chapter four) the shoulders are carried slightly behind a line drawn vertically through the ear, but if the thoracic spine is curved forwards, not only is the head carried well forward of this line (with a consequent additional extension of the neck being required to place the head in the normal position), but the shoulders tend to be carried even further forwards than the degree of spinal curvature might predict. This is due to a forward movement of the shoulder blades on the rib cage caused not only by the shapes and angles of the structures involved, but by the shortening of the muscles which pull the shoulders forward. Here a structural change is reinforced by muscular changes. To correct this, the spine needs to be encouraged to straighten slightly, and the shoulders to move backwards. This is achieved by stretching the shoulder muscles on the front of the body (including the chest muscles) and strengthening the muscles which pull the shoulders back. The following exercise affects this latter aspect and strengthens muscle groups involved in waist rotation.

Look at the photographs. The starting position looks like a single-arm dumbbell rowing movement. The weight is held by one arm, and the body's weight is supported on a bench by the other arm, which should be close to vertical under the shoulder. Ideally, the back is close to horizontal (to encourage the widest distribution of forces, and thus the most diffuse strengthening effect) and the leg opposite the arm holding the weight is bent and brought close to underneath the supporting arm (alternatively, you can kneel on this knee, although this variation is not shown). Let the weight pull the shoulder down (forwards to the floor) to the fullest extent.

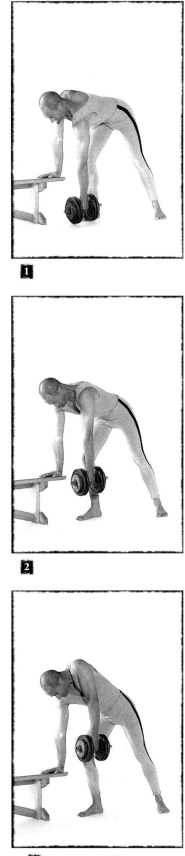

1

2

3

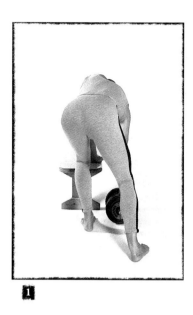

2

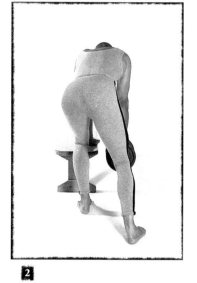

1

The movement is performed by using the waist and back muscles to lift the hanging shoulder as high as possible, **without** bending the arm at the elbow. However, the shoulder is pulled as far as possible towards the middle of the back. This action strongly involves the muscles which pull the shoulder back towards the spine (*rhomboid minor* and *major;* see illustration for exercise 8). Ensure that every part of the rotation of the shoulder is caused by muscular contraction and not by momentum—it is easy to cheat yourself in this movement.

Perform ten repetitions or so on one side first. After a suitable rest, repeat for the other side. Hold the finish position (the point of maximum rearward shoulder rotation) for a second or so at the end of each repetition. Breathe in at the same time during each repetition (to help develop a rhythm). The precise timing of breathing in the range of movement is not critical.

3

47. Lying rotations

This movement helps strengthen the waist muscles, but is much stronger than the previous exercise and works through a wider range of movement. This is also an excellent stretching exercise, since the maximum effect of the weight is experienced at the extremes of the range of the movement.

Begin your first attempt at this exercise with a light weight (for women 5 kg; for men 5–10 kg), holding it at arms' length as shown. Imagine that the weight is a mirror—as you do the movement, imagine that you are trying to watch your face. If you are able to do this, you will be able to maintain the weight and your chest in the correct relationship. Because we are handling the weight to strengthen the *waist* muscles, it is essential that every increment of movement at the hands is due to a rotation of the waist rather than a movement of the arms and shoulders with respect to the body. Think of the exercise in this way: the arms and chest form a rectangle with the weight, and this complex (weight, arms, chest) is moved as one, and moved by the waist and back muscles. Consider the photographs carefully—these details are important if you want to gain maximum benefit from the exercise.

Hold the weight, and visualise rotating only at the waist. Let the weight (together with the arms and chest) move across and sink towards the floor, slowly. If you are successful in not letting the arms move with respect to the chest, your shoulders will be close to vertical if you are flexible enough to lower the weight to the floor. Feel the stretch. Ideally, this should be felt in the muscles of the lower back, on the side you are turning away from (the upper side). Being aware of where you feel the stretch, slowly lift the weight back to the starting position using the stretched muscles.

The first few times you do the movement, go from one side to the other in turn, comparing sides. Do not be surprised if you find that they are not symmetrical. Asymmetry is common, and something one expects to find, particularly in people with back problems. Asymmetry comes in two basic forms in this movement: one side less flexible, or one side weaker. By experimenting (or in the light of other evidence

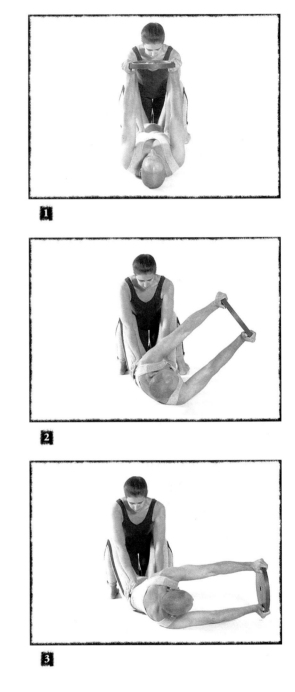

1

2

3

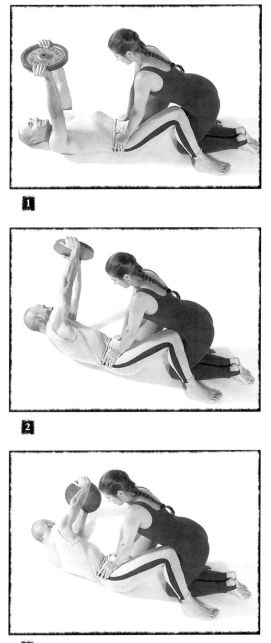

1

2

3

discussed below), choose which imbalance you wish to address.

The way to redress any imbalance is first to determine which side is the less flexible or the weaker. The next time you do the exercise, work only on that side to begin with. Let us say, for argument's sake, that you were able to do nine repetitions in good form on the weak (or tighter) side. Repeat the exercise now on the stronger or more flexible side, but do only as many repetitions as you were able to do for the first side. Doing so will be easier of course. The effect over time will be to stress the weaker or tighter side more than the other, so that it will respond more quickly. In enough time, the *functional* symmetries will become closer. Eventually they will be similar if not the same (for an amplification of this notion of functional versus structural symmetry, see chapter four). As a general rule, for any exercise one can do for one side of the body, the upper limit of repetitions or weight handled should be the same as what can be handled by the weaker or less flexible side.

48. Asymmetric weighted abdominal crunches

The floor version of the crunch (exercise 38 above) can be altered to produce an additional effect as with the asymmetric knee lifts outlined above (exercise 42). In this version, the resistance weight is held against one shoulder and the curling movement is performed towards the opposite hip. This means that in addition to the abdominal muscles at the front of the trunk, the obliques and the rib muscles on one side are also affected. The exercise should be done twice; the second time with the weight on the other shoulder. Because the abdominal muscles work wherever the weight is positioned, start the exercise with the weight on one shoulder one session, and on the other shoulder in the next exercise session. Over time, the net effect will be balanced. Although shown on the floor, this movement may also be done on an inclined board, affecting the lower abdominal muscles to a greater degree.

This completes the elements of my approach to overcoming neck and back pain. Let us now turn our attention to the integration of these various elements.

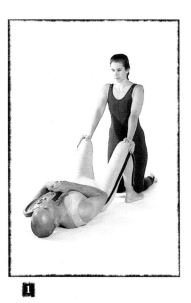

1

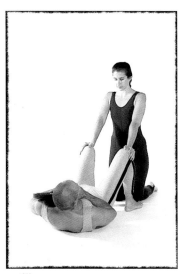

2

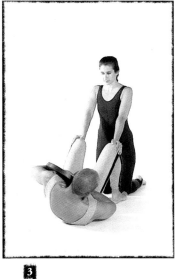

3

PLANNING A TOTAL ROUTINE

Frequency of exercise

You do not need to do anywhere near as much exercise as most experts say. Most people who start an exercise program abandon it within a month or six weeks. The main reason for this is that they have embarked on a program that is far too ambitious for their needs or (perhaps more significantly) their capacity. For a program to endure, and to be enjoyable—an essential aspect for any long-term prospects—it must fit your lifestyle. Moreover, despite the near-crippling exercise regimens your favourite athlete grinds through each day or week, your needs are not the same. Our goal is to optimise health, with an emphasis on rectifying, or preventing, neck and back pain.

Having said this, two Australian National women rowers I once coached trained with weights only twice a week for 30–40 minutes a session. This was complemented by two 10–15 minute stretching sessions each week, the stretching being done after the weight training. Their training involved only one set of each of seven exercises, some of these requiring a warm-up set. Each set was performed to complete failure; that is, until they were temporarily incapable of further repetitions, or even partial repetitions, of the movement. Their performance over a twelve-month period (as measured by ergometer) improved faster than that of their fellow crew-members, all of whom were doing three one-hour weight training sessions a week, each involving the usual three to five maximum sets, but with no stretching.

The point of this story is that the *quality* of your training is a far more significant determinant of improvement than is the amount of weight handled, the numbers of 'sets' and 'reps', or the total amount of work done. Nautilus Foundation researchers have demonstrated that the old adage 'less is more' is correct, as far as weight training is concerned, *provided* there is genuine maximum intensity. In conventional training the maximum intensity the body experiences with respect to any exercise usually occurs during the final few repetitions of the last set. If the research into determinants of adaptation is correct, the body responds to the stimulation of just those repetitions—any *previous* sets' repetitions (just because you were not exhausting yourself doing them) are more or less a waste of time.

In controlled tests, the amount of work done or the total amount of weight lifted in a session correlated less well with actual measured results of strength increases than the athlete's own subjective assessments of the intensity of the experience. Thus, providing the athlete worked to failure, the actual weights handled on any given day were not as significant in predicting strength gains over time. You are stronger on some days than on others—and on a weaker day, a smaller weight handled to failure seems to provoke the same adaptation as a heavier weight handled on a day when you feel stronger.

The multiple set approach of most weight training should be avoided for a number of reasons. Firstly, if you know that there are three or five maximum sets to be done, you cannot help saving yourself for following sets. This has two consequences. The first is that maximum intensity is experienced either in only one of the sets (in which case the others were a waste of time), or not experienced at all. Instead, you tend to work at about 80% of your possible capacity, doing a lot of work, but at sub-optimal intensity. This is commonly observed in gyms everywhere. The second consequence is that any sets not experienced at your maximum merely use energy and nutrients that otherwise would be used to repair the body after the maximum-intensity set. This implies strongly that sets before or additional to the one at which the maximum intensity was experienced actually *detract* from the training response. Furthermore, if you leave the gym knowing that you have worked at your maximum intensity yet also feeling that you have not exhausted yourself (that, in fact, you could do more work), your attitude to returning to the gym is positive and there is far less likelihood of overtraining or staleness. Overtraining is a real danger, even for the weekend athlete. Faster progress in strength training goals will be realised if the suggested approach is followed. The approach is much more efficient in terms of results gained for time spent. It is certainly more enjoyable.

The intensity of the experience seems to be the most important factor. Thus some specific recommendations can be made for your workouts, realising that individual requirements or reactions will alter the details in each case. Indeed, the shape and emphasis of your routine should change over time to reflect changing priorities and your improvement.

Sets and reps

The number of times you repeat a movement is referred to as the number of repetitions, or 'reps'. Groups of repetitions (from beginning to when you can do no more) are referred to as 'sets'. How many sets, of how many reps, should one do? Before making a specific recommendation, let us explore the standard approaches.

The conventional suggestions range from a standard of three sets of about ten repetitions to the serious bodybuilder's eight to twenty sets, with the repetitions varying from five to eight (or from ten to fifteen), depending on the desired outcome. For a bodybuilder, the choice is said to depend on whether one is working in a strengthening phase (to put on muscle weight) or a refining phase (to bring out the shape of muscles). Others suggest that the number of sets and repetitions depends on whether you are seeking strength or endurance. Strength is said to be achieved by larger numbers of low-repetition sets (for example, ten sets of three to five reps), and endurance by smaller numbers of sets, but with much higher repetitions (for example, three sets of 25 to 35 repetitions, common among rowers).

However, my suggestions are different. If you have a need to demonstrate maximum one-repetition strength levels (as with a competitive weightlifter, for example) then you need to follow a program which develops maximum strength in the whole structure and enables you to become familiar with handling weights which are close to your maximum for psychological and technical reasons. The dangers are obvious—the closer one is working to one's limit, the harder the exercise is to control, and the greater the possibility of injury. For this last reason alone, the maximum strength developing regime is not suitable for most of us. Neither is the high repetition endurance system, but for different reasons. We are not particularly interested in developing specific muscle endurance. This type of training is also relatively tiring, and the high repetitions do not help you concentrate on perfect form, which you will recall is the top priority. This approach is also obviously unsuitable for anyone suffering from any kind of repetitive strain injury.

The Nautilus Foundation derived an empirical approach to determining the ideal number of repetitions to promote muscle growth, but the method presupposes considerable experience with weight training. First you need to determine your one-repetition maximum (RM) lift in a particular exercise. For an experienced trainer this presents no special difficulty, but it is not appropriate for us. Nevertheless, to illustrate the approach, let us say that an athlete can do one all-out repetition of an exercise in good form with a weight of 100 kg. In the Nautilus method the athlete uses 80% of the RM (here, 80 kg) at a subsequent training session to do as many repetitions as possible. This number of repetitions becomes the number the athlete uses in his or her all-out maximum-effort sets in the routine, using the 80% RM weight. The RM test is repeated periodically, and the 80% RM weight adjusted as necessary. Perhaps paradoxically, athletes with a lower repetition count at 80% RM have a greater capacity to become stronger that those who can do more repetitions at 80%. This may indicate a smaller proportion of those muscle fibres that perform endurance tasks better, and hence a higher proportion of the fibres that limit ultimate strength. Although this method has some attraction, it is obviously unsuitable for beginners or those with injuries.

Because most of our exercises are done with the body's weight, the recommendations about selection of weight to be handled may seem somewhat academic. However, the principles as they relate to creation of the intensity effect remain relevant, and most can be implemented directly.

Taking account of the research on the different sets and reps approaches, it is best to err on the side of caution, and attempt an exercise with a lighter weight than you imagine you might be able to handle, and concentrate on attaining good form. *Good form must always remain the first priority.* As mentioned, in some of the exercises, you may not be able to do even one repetition with your body's weight—if so, get your partner to help and do the negative version. I recommend only one set of each exercise.

When you can do 15 repetitions of the movement, increase the weight—but only to one which permits a *minimum* of eight repetitions. The initial repetitions in the set will constitute a sufficient warm-up, but the final four or five repetitions will be at maximum effort. In body's weight exercises, the weight which you will add may be very light and yet provide a significant additional resistance. For example, if you initially do the hanging knee lifting movement without shoes, it will take some time before you can do 15 repetitions. When that day comes, do the exercise with your shoes on next time. Although relatively light, the addition of this weight makes a significant difference, because of the leverage factors (the length of thighs).

However, even following this prescription will not provide the ideal intensity for some exercises. How then can you follow the prescription and further increase intensity? The answer is to add *resistance reduction*, *assisted repetitions*, *negative repetitions* and *partial repetitions* to your one set, singly or in combination.

Resistance reduction means that you reduce the weight by a small amount as soon as you feel that you will be unable to complete another full repetition without assistance. For example, assume that you are doing a barbell exercise with 30 kg. Thinking ahead, you will have made this weight up with two 10 kg plates, and two 5 kg plates. As soon as you feel that you are failing or losing the form, put the weight back on the stands. Ask your partner to take the two 5 kg plates off and recommence the exercise at once. These weight recommendations are a guide only—depending on the exercises you will need to have the increments smaller or larger. This approach can be applied to body's weight exercises (once you are using extra weight) by dropping the weight when you have tired, and continuing with body weight alone.

Assisted repetitions are another way to prolong the repetitions at maximum effort. They can be used with either concentric or eccentric movements. Some exercises lend themselves to this technique in virtue of their physical arrangements—assistance is easier to give in some exercises than others. For example, to assist in the hanging knee lift movement, your partner waits until you can no longer perform another movement in good form. Then (by placing his or her palms under your feet or supporting the front of the knees) your partner takes a small amount of the weight of your legs as you try to lift them. Even reducing the weight of your legs by a tiny amount will enable you to do more repetitions. After all, muscle failure occurs when the tension the muscles are capable of applying only *just* fails to overcome the resistance. Reducing the resistance by even a small amount can let the muscles continue to work. In this way, the point of imminent failure—which is the very intensity I have been stressing throughout—can be prolonged for five or more repetitions beyond the point at which you would have otherwise stopped.

The term *negative repetitions* (eccentric contractions, or negatives for short) was used previously when discussing how to do an exercise you could not do positively (concentrically). This approach can also be used to prolong the maximum effort phase of any exercise, after you have done as many repetitions as possible in the positive phase.

For example, assume you have done your non-assisted repetitions in the hanging knee lift exercise. Have your partner immediately lift your knees to your chest. Try to hold them there for an instant. As you feel yourself weakening, lower the knees slowly—a good negative repetition should take about four seconds—and fight the resistance all the way to the starting position. Again, before you have any chance to rest, have your partner lift your knees and let them go as soon as they reach your chest. Finish the exercise when you cannot prevent your knees from falling to the start position. Generally, this will require about five repetitions. This is very high intensity work indeed, so do not be in too much of a hurry to progress to this technique—it will leave the muscles very sore.

To experience the maximum in intensity, negative repetitions can even be added to an exercise after you have done a number of assisted repetitions (assisted in the positive phase) for an even greater effect. However, do not attempt this until you are completely confident with the assisted approach. Adding the negatives to the assisted method is extremely intense, and must not be attempted by anyone who has even a hint of their previous problems remaining.

Partial repetitions are unsuccessful attempts to complete full repetitions. The partial repetition that results is both isotonic (while the weight is still moving) and isometric (the point at which the weight no longer moves, no matter how hard you try). Partial repetitions can be used as a variation on combinations of the above elements, such as when you do not feel like progressing into the negative phases (for example, if you do not have a training partner, or do not feel like pushing yourself too hard). The hanging knee lift is a good example of an exercise that can be done in a variety of ways, by combining these different elements.

Working habits

As mentioned previously, many people begin training programs and give up after a short time. In addition to embarking on programs that are unsuitable or too ambitious, some of these people drop out because they fail to take into account personal lifestyle factors—such as children, or the demands of work. For example, it is impossible to do your stretching exercises with your three-year-old child crawling all over you, and very unlikely that you will even feel like exercising after a 14-hour day at work. Part of the success of any exercise program is to choose the right time and the right location for your exercise, and not to take on too much.

The best time to stretch is in the late afternoon or evening before you have your evening meal, when the body is at its loosest. Although strengthening exercises can be done at any time, for someone getting over an injury it is best to avoid the mornings because the body is at its tightest. However, if you are a morning person, and you warm up carefully, then (presupposing that you are injury-free) begin with the strengthening exercises and finish with the stretching exercises. Avoid doing strengthening exercises at night too soon before you sleep because they tend to stimulate the body and this may affect your sleep.

Any strength training (or aerobic training) is a perfect warm-up for stretching—just try to keep as much of the generated body heat in the muscles by wearing the appropriate clothes. The secret to maintaining a successful program is to integrate it as seamlessly as possible into *your* normal routine.

If time constraints (or children) make these suggestions impracticable, you can still do the stretching exercises on the lounge room floor while watching television—after the children have gone to bed. Alternatively, it is a lot of fun to do these exercises with your children if they are old enough—and it is never too early to teach good habits.

Speed of movements

The correct speed of movement is critical. We have already considered the speed of stretching and must now look at the speed of strengthening exercises.

In the positive phase of any movement, each increment of movement of the resistance weight—whether an object or part of your body—must be achieved by muscular contraction, and not by momentum generated in an earlier part of the movement. This cannot be overemphasised, and is second only to the importance of form. Do not make the movements too slow, either. As a rough guide (remembering that this will depend on the nature of the exercise to an extent), a positive contraction exercise should take about two to three seconds to complete, and negatives about twice as long.

Do not pause too long in either the extended or contracted phase of a movement. Usually, the beginning or end points of an exercise are relatively easy to hold and as such provide a rest for the muscles. Remember that we are trying to fatigue the muscles in the *shortest* possible time, and that prolonging the exercise defeats this goal. Try to put your total concentration into each instant of the doing of an exercise—this increases its intensity and reduces the chance of injury.

The importance of rest

Do not train too much. All adaptation to stimulation occurs *after* training, not during it. Accordingly, to adapt as fast as possible you will need to ensure that you have adequate rest. Studies show that all stress causes effects in the body—good and bad stress—and that the effects of one kind of stress tend to compound with those of other kinds of stress. These studies also show that everyone has an innate capacity to handle stress, and that if this capacity is exceeded the body cannot adapt to new stress.

As far as the body is concerned, a new exercise program is just another stress. Examples of stress include your job (the stress of which is likely to vary, depending on what you are doing at any time), other training you may be involved in, or any significant change to your normal routine. Accordingly, you may need to reduce your involvement in other stressing activities if you wish to adapt to the new stress as quickly as possible.

The place of aerobic exercise

Swimming is often recommended to help alleviate back pain. This recommendation is usually made on the assumption that, because swimming is an aerobic activity in which the body's weight is supported while it is horizontal, it is good for patients recovering or suffering from back pain. My experience with this recommendation runs counter to the generalisation. My reasons are to do with the *style* of swimming adopted by the patient. If the patient is a good freestyle swimmer, the recommendation is generally sound, and the gentle and supported flexion and extension of the spine yields beneficial results. This may be the result of a mechanical effect on the intervertebral discs that increases water imbibition by the disc nucleus and helps to restore disc height.

However, if the patient is not a good freestyle swimmer, and has to use breast stroke or another style, swimming can exacerbate problems. This is the result of the slight-to-moderate hyperextension of the lumbar spine, and the contraction in the back muscles required to hold the head out of the water. For the same reasons, in cases of neck pain this problem can be significant. Many patients with back problems have reported that swimming makes their complaints worse. Thus swimming should not be used early in the rehabilitation phase, unless you are a good swimmer and the activity does not irritate the problem. However, swimming is excellent aerobic activity that can help to keep back pain at bay—once the back has returned to normal.

Running is also an excellent aerobic activity, but has obvious drawbacks for sufferers of back pain. The whole weight of the body is carried on the legs, there can be some slight-to-significant compression of the lumbar region, there are mechanical shocks to the spine with each step, and most people run on hard surfaces that tend to exacerbate these problems. These negative aspects are worsened if the patient is carrying excess body weight. If the.

patient is a long-term runner, there is also a strong likelihood that the muscles of the lower back, the groin, and the hamstrings will be less flexible than average, and this also tends to exacerbate the back pain. The importance of leg-length differences cannot be over-emphasised. In general, a person suffering from back pain should not run until the pain has reduced to a non-significant level.

Cycling can be quite comfortable for the sufferer of back pain. However, it is contraindicated for the patient with neck pain, depending on the style of cycling. Racing bikes place a strain on the back of the neck and the upper back, whereas mountain bikes generally deliver more road shock to the lower back but place less strain on the neck, due to the more upright riding position. The value in cycling, especially stationary cycling, is that you can effectively and safely warm-up the muscles you need to stretch. If you wear the appropriate clothes you can retain much of this heat. Remember that an increase of just one degree in core muscle temperature can increase flexibility 15% or more, and when your body is tight every fraction of a per cent of flexibility is significant.

Other values in aerobic activity during the recovery phase include the general feeling of well being after exercise. This helps orient oneself to an optimistic frame of mind and maintain your desired body weight. Both are critical to a successful recovery.

Lifting things in everyday life

Before ending this chapter on strengthening techniques, we should look at how to avoid injuries while lifting. The most common history of patients with acute back pain, and the most common prelude to disc prolapse, is an unexceptional lifting movement done around the house or workplace that combines *extension* with *rotation*. No such movement has been included in the strengthening exercises presented, with good reason.

A typical movement that combines rotation with extension is to pick up a garbage can which *is on the ground to one side of you*. You not only bend forwards, but also rotate to one side. To pick the can up, you must lift with the legs and twist with the waist muscles. This can place large, unsymmetrical forces on both the intervertebral discs (especially the one between the last vertebra and the sacrum) and on the muscles of the lower back (*quadratus lumborum*). These forces may tear the muscles or force the disc to extrude—both extremely painful outcomes.

Consider the Olympic and powerlifting movements (the 'clean' and the 'deadlift'), wherein very heavy weights are lifted. These movements take advantage of the body's great strength when used efficiently—that is, when forces applied to it are distributed as widely as possible. This can occur only when all parts of the body involved in the movement can share the load. In the garbage can movement described, this is far from true. The lessons to be learned from this are simple. When picking anything up, the following rules must be observed:

- Directly face the object to be lifted;

- Bend the knees and minimise bending forwards from the hips;

- Hold the trunk as straight as you can (*if you cannot, the weight is too heavy for you to lift*);

- Have your weight evenly distributed through both hands and over both feet;

- Hold the object as close to the body as you can;

- Hold the object with straight arms, as far as practicable; and

- Take in a breath and hold it when performing the actual lifting movement.

Always focus your attention on what you are doing. This may seem like gratuitous advice, but most injuries occur when you are doing something physical while your attention is focused elsewhere. *Never* combine a lifting and twisting movement.

These remarks apply to the typical untrained individual. Obviously, a discus thrower or similar athlete can ignore this advice, because he or she has trained hard to be able to do just this movement. However, unless you are such a specialist athlete, you would be well advised to observe these rules. Olympic and powerlifters handle enormous weights in their events. If you observe them carefully, you will see that even they obey *all* of these rules, without exception. Perhaps surprisingly, back injuries are rarer in these sports than in most other track and field events, despite the huge stresses they impose on the lower back.

The daily six

A number of readers have pointed out that I did not include the exercises we call 'the daily six' from the *Posture & Flexibility* classes anywhere in the first edition of the book. The reason is that the intended audiences of the book and the classes are different, and that we do not use chairs in the class situation. However, since I decided to make the video tapes (which include two versions of the daily six, one for the neck and one for the back), I have decided to add a generic version here. The exercises I recommend be done daily are exercises 1 and 2 (here considered as one exercise), 8 (whichever version suits your proportion), 23 (whichever feels most comfortable), 9, 13 (version 2), and finish with exercise 3. Gentle C–R stretches can be done in all exercises except 23.

Pointers to chapter four, causes, and chapter five, relaxation techniques

Chapter four deals with the causes of neck and back pain, and is a little more technical than preceding chapters. Chapter five deals with a simple approach to learning how to relax. A great deal has been written on this subject, and the consensus of opinion is that, especially with neck and back pain, the development of relaxation habits (which can be learned quite easily) speeds up the healing process. *Applying* these lessons will be the more difficult matter, but the motivation that has carried you this far should help you prevail. If you wish, you may proceed to chapter five, and return to chapter four at a later time.

THE CAUSES OF NECK AND BACK PAIN

This chapter gives an overview of the causes of back pain, from the perspectives of a number of different kinds of medicine. Central to all forms of medicine is the notion of cause, and this concept is used as an organising theme for this chapter. The chapter explores some of the reasons why the very idea of cause can be a problem with respect to common illnesses like neck and back pain. The last part of this chapter is written for practitioners who deal with neck and back pain, and who may be interested in an expanded analysis of my structural–functional approach to these problems. Although written primarily for the practitioner, the general reader should also find much of interest.

The prevailing theories

Many researchers claim that humans are predisposed to back problems. One leading anatomist claims that the lumbar lordosis (the backward-facing concavity of the lower part of the spine, closest to the hips) is a major weakness of the body, due in part to the shearing forces present at the lumbosacral interface (that is, the joint between the fifth lumbar vertebra and the first sacral vertebra, L5–S1). Most back operations are performed at this junction.

Kapandji hypothesises that this potential weakness arises from the transition from quadrupedal to bipedal (four-legged to two-legged) movement in our distant evolutionary past. The human spine, which was originally a single curve anteriorly, became straight and then the lower part curved further backward to form the spine's present shape. According to some researchers, the normal lumbar lordosis is said to have resulted because the pelvis has not yet tilted far enough posteriorly. The same changes in curvature from anterior to posterior are observed during the first ten years of life; thus 'the phylogenic [evolutionary] changes are recapitulated during ontogeny [development]' (Kapandji, 1974, vol. III, p.16).

Henderson states that the lumbar spine of most quadrupedal vertebrates is a smooth anterior curve. Animals with a lordotic curve—such as dogs and horses—also suffer spinal problems. Thus, humans are 'predisposed to [certain kinds of] low back pathology' (1985, p.1156). Interestingly, a number of chiropractors specialise in treating horses and dogs for back problems.

However, there are also convincing arguments for a contrary position. The lumbar curve can also be seen as a superb adaptation mechanism—without its three curves (see the illustration for details) the spine would have almost no longitudinal shock-absorbing capacity, and every step would jar the skull. Film analysis has shown that when a person is walking or running the head hardly moves at all vertically, and most of the pelvic movement vertically is absorbed by the curves of the spine tightening and releasing. Moreover, engineering analyses have shown that the curves of the spine significantly increase its resistance to axial compression loads.

The argument of maladaptive evolutionary change does not explain why some people never suffer back pain. The arguments for and against humans being prone to back problems because of basic 'design' faults are equally convincing—or unconvincing. No overwhelmingly persuasive evidence exists for either position. A pragmatic position is that this is how we are, and that the arguments perhaps are of more interest to anatomists than those who wish to do something about the problem.

One theory of back weakness

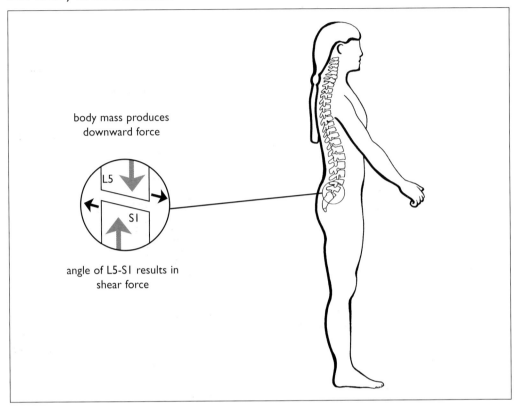

body mass produces
downward force

L5

S1

angle of L5-S1 results in
shear force

The three curves of the spinal column act as a shock absorber

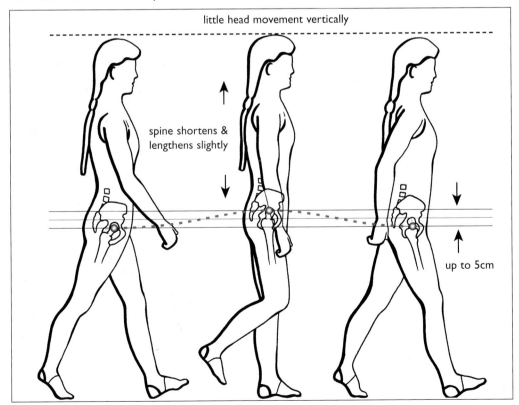

little head movement vertically

spine shortens &
lengthens slightly

up to 5cm

Schematic of spine, vertebral bodies and disc

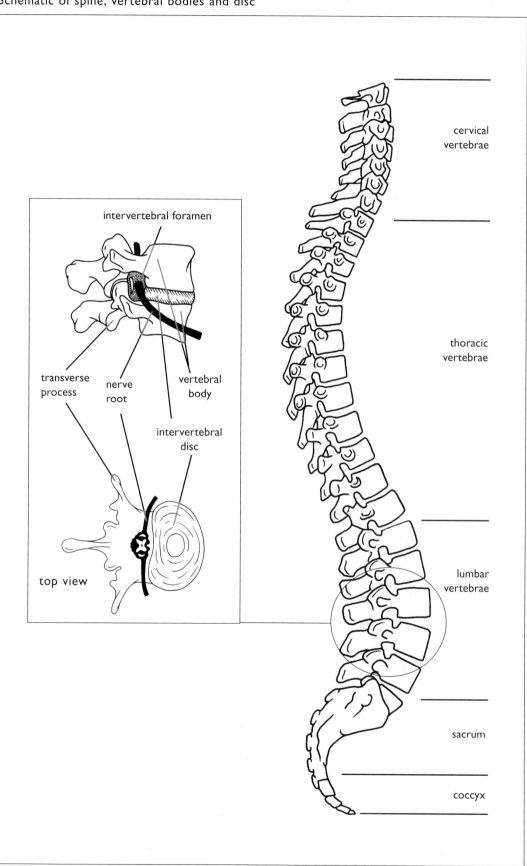

intervertebral foramen

transverse
process

nerve
root

vertebral
body

intervertebral
disc

top view

cervical
vertebrae

thoracic
vertebrae

lumbar
vertebrae

sacrum

coccyx

Nonetheless, the vertebral column has long been accepted by most doctors as the cause in the great majority of episodes of chronic back pain. As Ganora states 'there is little doubt that most cases are due to derangement of the intervertebral joint in association with "degeneration" of the disc and arthrosis of the facet joints.' In the following sentence he says 'Exactly which structures within this motion segment are the actual sources of pain remains conjectural' (Ganora, 1984, p.55).

Other researchers take a different view. Murtagh says that 'most back pain is minor, caused by ligamentous and muscular strains which usually subside without treatment; the general practitioner sees the more severe cases' (1983, p.322). He states that 'spinal derangement' accounted for over 67% of back pain in his survey of 1,000 patients. Expert opinion is divided over whether disc protrusion or 'overriding' of the pain sensitive apophyseal joints [or facet joints, the joints between the vertebrae] is the cause (Murtagh, 1983).

Fifty years ago, a paper published by Mixter and Barr provided the theoretical foundation and justification for a wave of back operations over the next two decades, described by one commentator as 'the dynasty of the disc' (Henderson, 1985). This early paper first used the term 'intervertebral disc lesion', often called a 'slipped' disc in common usage. The term refers to the partial or complete extrusion of the soft, gelatinous centre (nucleus) of the intervertebral disc, which are the 'cushions' of shock-absorbing material separating pairs of vertebrae.

During the 1940s and 1950s, many exploratory laminectomies (operations that partly or completely excise disc material) were performed with indifferent results (Henderson, 1985), illustrating the connection between theory and practice. One researcher claimed that this 'mammoth surgical exercise' was inevitable, because the solution appeared simple—removal of the disc would cure the problem (Taylor, cited by Twomey, 1974). As is now well accepted, this was not the case. However, even today the accepted wisdom at the first point of contact most patients have with the medical profession—the general practitioner—is that some kind of disc or vertebral problem is the most likely cause of acute or chronic back pain.

If one does not go to a general practitioner for a neck or a back problem, the next most likely recourse will be to a chiropractor or an osteopath. Chiropractic and osteopathy both rely on a particular 'lesion' of the spine as the main cause of back pain. They use the term 'subluxation', which is defined as 'a clinically significant disturbance of joint movement or position which responds to manipulation' (Charlton, 1988). The Macquarie Dictionary describes a subluxation as a 'partial dislocation' (Macquarie, 1981). Treatment consists of 'long leverage mobilisation techniques' (osteopaths) or 'short leverage dynamic thrust techniques' (chiropractors), which are said to restore normal function to the joint in question (Bolton, 1987).

Generally, the ministrations of osteopaths are more gentle than those of chiropractors, and involve a preparatory massage of the area to be manipulated. However, the differences between the two practices seem to be dwindling and cross-fertilisation of techniques is common. One chiropractor considered the differences between the practice of different chiropractors at least as significant as the putative differences between the two professions.

It is of some concern that the subluxation both professions rely on has never been 'proved' as an 'independently verifiable, clinically significant entity' (Charlton, 1988). It needs to be said here that 'proved', in this context, means proved to the satisfaction of the orthodox western medical profession. Obviously, chiropractors and osteopaths themselves have no problem with the concept in either theory or practice, nor do most of their large number of patients. This finding may have more to do with the standards of evidence being applied to the problem than any shortcomings in the techniques—that is, it may be the case that the standards of proof being sought are unreasonably restrictive. There is little doubt that many people gain relief from their problems through chiropractic and osteopathic techniques.

Oriental medicine is also used to treat back pain. The approach is based on an understanding of the body that differs significantly from that of western scientific medicine that provides the basis of orthodox medicine, chiropractic and osteopathy. The latter treatments have allied themselves with western medicine in Australia only quite recently, following a pattern of discrimination similar to that seen in both the United States and Great Britain in earlier times. In Australia, all recent chiropractic and osteopathic practitioners have an appropriate Bachelor of Applied Science degree from one of the major metropolitan universities.

In contrast to the biological–physical (biophysical) approach of western medicine, oriental medicine is based on a distinctly different cosmology. The oriental systems postulate a flow of energy (*chi* or *ki*) around the body through fourteen channels called meridians—lines of energy which flow around the body connecting the familiar acupuncture points. Disruptions to the normal flow of energy are considered to be the cause of disease (including illnesses like back pain), and accordingly an approach aimed at re-balancing this flow is used to help the problem. Treatment uses manual pressure, needles, or heat applied to the acupuncture points judged to be effective in restoring this balance. Interestingly, it is common that such practitioners are as likely to treat areas far removed from the site of the patient's complaint as the area itself. In cases of back pain, the determination of the cause of the problem is normally made with reference to disturbances to meridians rather than to the structures of the back itself.

The oriental systems can also avail themselves of various exercise forms. However, in contrast to physiotherapy or the like, the exercise is not explicitly to stretch or strengthen the muscles involved, but is more indirect. Practitioners of oriental medicine usually claim that the purpose of the exercise is to restore a desirable energy flow.

Acute pain

Western medicine is at its best treating the sort of back pain that results from acute trauma, such as a car accident. Acute trauma (for example, a compression injury that might crush particular discs) can be extremely dangerous, with a risk of partial or complete paralysis if left untreated. Such paralysis is generally caused by mechanical compression of segmental nerves, which exit from the spinal column between pairs of vertebrae. (This condition is often referred to as 'nerve impingement'.) Surgery is used to relieve the pressure on the nerves, and sometimes bone grafts are used to stabilise the pairs of vertebrae involved.

Posterolateral *(back-side)* extrusion of intervertebral disc impinging on nerve root

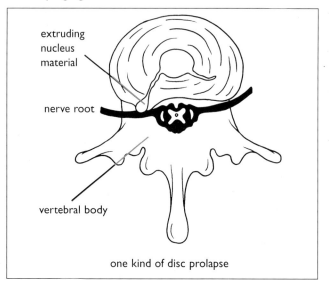

extruding nucleus material

nerve root

vertebral body

one kind of disc prolapse

The precise site of the injury can be inferred from the location of what are called 'neurological deficits'. This term refers to patterns of loss of sensation, tingling in the muscles of the legs or feet, or loss of movement in specific muscle groups. Maps of the body called 'dermatome charts' show the relationships between particular muscles and their innervating nerves. These charts are used to identify the involved nerve and hence the site of the damage. However, this kind of acute segmental nerve impingement accounts for less than 5% of cases of acute back pain. The most important question to answer is whether neurological signs exist—if they do, seek the assistance of your family doctor.

Another common cause of neck or back pain is associated with acute muscle spasm, although one researcher claims that 'there is no scientific evidence that muscles are a primary cause of lumbar spine pain' (Saal, 1988). If the spasm is located in the neck muscles, the condition is known as *torticollis* (Latin for 'twisted neck') or perhaps more familiarly, a wry neck. Muscle spasm is a strong, involuntary muscular contraction that you are unable to relax. The cause of such a condition is sometimes unclear—it may be the precursor to a cold or a bout of the 'flu, sleeping near an open window, or the result of unaccustomed activity. If the latter, the condition probably results from very small-scale lesions ('micro-trauma', or small ruptures) to the muscle fibres themselves, causing a vigorous contraction of the surrounding fibres that may be an involuntary protective mechanism to prevent further injury.

If a similar micro-trauma is responsible for an episode of acute back pain (particularly likely if you suspect that unaccustomed activity is the cause), take heart in the statistics. No matter how agonising in the first instance, more than half such patients are better within a week, and more than 85% recover within three weeks. The best figures available (compiled from the authors listed in the reference section) suggest that after two months, fewer than 3% have any ongoing problems. Most general practitioners used to advise bed-rest, but active rest is now the more common recommendation. Active rest usually involves avoiding the activity judged to be primarily responsible, and often includes advice to seek physiotherapy or massage. A less frequent cause of acute pain may be an internal problem such as a urinary tract or kidney infection. Occasionally, muscle spasm results from disc prolapse (which can be accompanied by sciatica) or from partial or complete fractures of the vertebrae. Further consideration of another possible cause of sciatica is made at the end of this chapter.

Chronic pain

It is commonly accepted that most people will suffer back pain on some occasion in life. The main reason that people regard back pain so seriously is that when it occurs it is completely debilitating. A pulled muscle in the arm or leg is certainly inconvenient, and perhaps even painful, but many of life's normal activities can continue until the injury heals. As anyone who has suffered can attest, this is not the case with back pain—one's whole life, in its smallest and largest parts, is affected.

How much worse, then, is the plight of the sufferer of chronic back pain? All aspects of life are affected to some degree—work, relationships, and recreational activities. The main focus of this book is chronic back pain and its alleviation. Before considering possible predisposing factors, one important question to be answered is whether your chronic pain continues unremittingly through the night. If this is the case, discuss the condition with your doctor to eliminate possible malignancies. Malignancy is the cause of back pain in about 1% of patients (Murtagh, 1985).

Loss of disc height is commonly offered as an explanation for chronic back pain. The theory is that, as 'normal' wear and tear to the intervertebral discs occurs, the discs lose some of their thickness. As mentioned previously, the segmental nerves exit the spine from the spinal cord through a space created by pairs of notches in adjoining vertebrae, not through fixed 'holes'. In the normal individual, there is enough space between the various structures—including the disc, a number of ligaments, and the dura (the sheath of the spinal cord through which the nerve must exit)—for normal bending of the spine in any of its directions to have no ill effects.

However, these spaces become narrower as disc height is lost. Very little height needs to be lost before the surrounding structures apply pressure to the segmental nerves, causing pain at the site of the pressure, and sometimes pain at more distant locations (referred pain). Loss of disc height may also result in increased pressure on the facet joints, the sliding joints of the vertebrae, which are rich in nerves. Loss of disc height can also cause familiar sciatica (literally, pain in the sciatic nerve). Although this explanation may account for the primary cause in the extreme case, it is unlikely to be the whole explanation. Even sufferers of chronic back pain have good days, with little or no pain. Other factors besides vertebral pathology must also play a causal role.

One contributing cause is tension held in the muscles surrounding the site of the original injury. Tension increases in muscles surrounding any kind of physical trauma. The tension is a protective mechanism, to limit further injury to an area by limiting its movement. If the tension is held for a long time (from weeks to years) a number of effects are noticed. One is that the protective tension becomes a habit, in effect reinforcing the original problem. A 'feedback loop' is set up between the muscle fibres and the central nervous system, so that the pain signals cause a re-stimulation of the contracting fibres. If this continues, it may be accompanied by systemic changes to the relationship between the nerves and the muscle fibres, until (to continue the computer metaphors) the pain–contraction condition becomes 'hard-wired' into the system. If this occurs, the resulting changes are known by various names like *fibrosis*. Collagen is deposited in the area, forming hard knots in the affected muscles. If this condition is left untreated, the condition can become very difficult to change.

During healing following an injury, collagen fibres (long strings of protein) are laid down in a random pattern. Electron microscope photographs show that the resulting fibres run in all directions initially. Over time, the fibres align themselves in response to forces applied to them. The crucial lesson is that knots in muscles following injury, or the often dramatic reduction in range of movement often observed after trauma, can result from healing itself. If the new collagen is not stressed in a way that mimics the demands of normal life, the affected muscle will have a reduced range of movement. Stress drives adaptation. For this reason, to restore normal function, it is essential to stretch an injured part (very carefully, initially) and then strengthen it.

Another possible effect, without any detectable *physiological* change in the tissues involved, is that a particular pattern or way of holding the body may result—a 'postural signature'. Such a pattern may be as difficult to change as a more physiologically-based change. For example, consider someone who has had a broken leg in plaster for about six weeks. When the plaster is removed and physiotherapy has re-established the previous size, strength and tone of the leg, a patient may still walk in a way that favours the leg. This altered movement pattern can persist for months or even years and can be extremely difficult to alter.

Emotional factors also play a role in chronic neck or back pain. The distinction between the physical and the mental becomes less clear the closer one looks at the way the whole body works. Nonetheless, the distinction is useful, providing one realises that it is made for our convenience. Emotional factors refer to a range of attitudes and behaviours, from a more-or-less conscious choice to remove oneself from an undesirable situation by becoming ill (hence legitimating the absence) to normal reactions to stress or fatigue. Although not as directly obvious a cause as a trauma, the effects may well be as debilitating, and must be considered in treatment.

The great psychotherapist Wilhelm Reich coined the term 'character armour' to describe the tendency of the injured child to accrete protective layers that, if left untreated, become the protective armour experienced (and displayed) by the adult. By armour, he referred to the great range of emotional or behavioural problems afflicting adults. Such armour has the well-known advantage of protection, but at the cost of rigidity and pain. He concluded that trauma experienced by the psyche manifests itself at the physical level of experience as tightness in the muscles, organ dysfunction, and pain. One of his solutions was a form of massage. Central to his approach to curing a patient's problem was restoration of normal physical function. Reich believed that returning the body's function to normal also healed the original injury to the psyche—'stored' in the tissues of the body—so that the complaint did not return.

Other contributing factors

The picture presented so far may have given the impression that any deformation to the body's symmetry is caused by some kind of trauma. This is not the case. It is well accepted in western medicine that a condition named the *short-leg syndrome* exists. This condition is said to exist when one leg is more than nine millimetres shorter than its fellow. Although we assume that our bodies are symmetrical, this may not be the case. We need to determine exactly at which point a deviation from symmetry is likely to become significant. If it were easy to measure, a one millimetre difference in leg length would not normally be judged significant. Why the nine millimetre threshold was chosen is not clear, and in some individuals smaller differences can also be significant. For example, if the nine millimetre threshold is significant for a 185 cm male, a lesser difference will produce an identical tilting of the pelvis of a 150 cm male (as measured in degrees from horizontal) if his hips are narrower than the taller person's (see the illustration).

Like many of the determinations of medicine, this threshold applies in the general case to the average person—a statistical entity. The additional complicating factor is the question

Schematic showing significance of leg-length difference

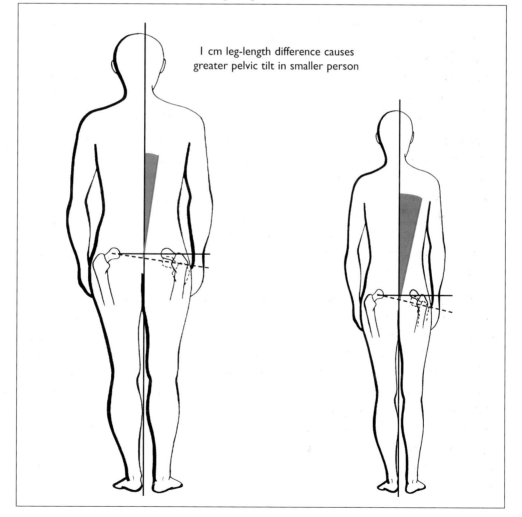

1 cm leg-length difference causes greater pelvic tilt in smaller person

of whether the observed short leg is structural (the leg bones of one leg being shorter than the other) or induced. The latter can occur as an adaptation to a scoliosis (lateral curvature of the spine), through tension held in particular muscles for a variety of reasons, or shortness in muscles due to previous injury.

Other structural problems may be seen by looking at the body from the side. For example, there may be an exaggerated curve of the upper spine *(kyphosis)*, or of the lower back (lordosis). Kyphosis is always accompanied by an exaggerated extension of the neck (a backwards arching), which becomes necessary to hold the head level. This structural condition alone can produce strong tension in the muscles needed to hold the head in this position. It is safe to say that any deviation from a posited 'ideal' will require some compensatory adaptation from another part. It is generally accepted in engineering theory that the maximum strength of any structure is achieved by the widest distribution of forces throughout the whole structure. Patients with a structural problem always have increased tension in particular muscles—those required to do extra work to support the body's shape. These tighter areas almost always coincide with the loci of pain.

Asymmetry in the balances between flexibility and strength in various areas around the body can also produce deviations from the ideal. It is useful sometimes to consider strength as a lack of flexibility—or to consider flexibility as being equivalent to insufficient strength—due to the relationship of these properties in forming the characteristic shape of the individual. For example, tight *psoas* and *iliacus* muscles (*iliopsoas,* the hip flexors) together can tilt the pelvis anteriorly, producing the familiar lumbar lordosis (sway back). This does not involve structural asymmetry or spinal abnormality. The excessive tension (strength) of these muscles is not balanced by an appropriate group, such as the abdominal muscles. Another way to consider the same problem is to assert that the *iliopsoas* muscles are insufficiently flexible. The reasons for making this distinction will become clearer when we see how the two concepts offer two different solutions.

Shortcomings with the idea of cause

We are used to the language of causality—that a particular effect is caused by something. Cause is familiar to us and pervades our way of thinking about the world. However, for the practitioner the usefulness of the ordinary idea of cause has many problems. It is even possible that the search for the cause of an illness may itself limit solutions.

Back pain is a good example of the problems of establishing the relation between symptom and cause. Western medicine considers vertebral pathology to be the main cause of back pain. Here, 'pathology' is used as shorthand for a range of deviations from normal, from abnormalities of the vertebrae to disease of the vertebral structures. However, radiography reveals degenerative change in the vertebral structures of most people over 30 years old, and about one fifth of this population never suffers back pain (Laughlin, 1989). As mentioned, epidemiological studies suggest that about half of the patients suffering acute back pain at any time are well within a week and over 85% are well within a month. However, vertebral pathology does not change significantly within these time frames. Confounding the issues are the results of a unique study published in the *New England Journal of Medicine* (Jensen *et al.,* 1994). Using MRI (magnetic resonance imaging) technology, the researchers found that two-thirds of a group studied had the sort of abnormalities or disease which would be judged as the cause of pain had they been found in a back pain sufferer—yet the group had been selected from a sample of people who never had back pain.

The inconsistency in these results may be explained by suggesting that pathology exists benignly until other factors make it significant. However, because of medicine's desire to establish causal chains, diagnostic procedures designed to reveal the presence of pathology are employed. If pathology is found, back pain will be attributed to it (Laughlin, 1989).

However, there are two problems in tracing cause in this common illness. The first problem is that back pain is widely described in the literature as having a 'multifactorial aetiology' (many causal factors). The answer to the question of whether a potential cause should be considered cumulative, passive, or even countervailing, with respect to other co-existing causes, is far from clear. The first difficulty is to determine which cause of the multiple possible causes is the most important. Rules such as Occam's razor (that one is bound to choose the simplest explanation which fits the evidence) provide a useful constraint for the practitioner.

The second problem is whether or not orthodox western medicine has a treatment for the particular cause identified. This problem suggests a practical relation between the ascription of 'pathology' (as a label for a cluster of characteristics) and the prescription of treatment. The relation also partly explains medicine's tendency to define illness in terms of those attributes of the problem which are identifiable by the current technology (such as radiology, MRI [magnetic resonance imaging], or CAT [computerised axial tomography] scans, for example) and basing treatment on the results.

Determining the cause of your problems is useful for both selecting and monitoring treatment. Which cause do you select? Considering our ongoing example, the short leg and its role in back pain, why do practitioners not focus attention on what might be *its* cause? And what of the cause that gave rise to it? In fact, every cause has a cause—how far back do you go in your analysis? This is one problem. Another is the problem of causes accompanying causes (the typical multifactorial or multi-causal illness)—which do you select for treatment? What is the relationship between these multiple causes? Do their effects compound, does one counteract another, or is one possible cause nullified by another cause? Let us consider the short-leg syndrome as an example.

When one leg is shorter than the other, the normal curves of the spine in the sagittal plane are subtly reproduced in the coronal plane (refer to the illustration overleaf). This adaptation to uneven loads on the pelvis enables us to balance, by distribution of the asymmetric forces produced around the sacrum. A person with a slightly shorter right leg (with consequent tilting of the pelvis), will thus carry his or her left shoulder on the outside of a gently rightward curving thoracic spine (as seen from behind) if no other factors are present. This lateral curve (accompanied by additional development of the muscles on its convex side) may be a *cumulating* cause of *neck* pain in a left-handed person or a *countervailing* cause in a right-handed person. This is because of the increased muscular development (and usually increased tension) of the *trapezius* and *levator scapulae* muscles on the side of the dominant arm. In a right-handed person, the effects of these asymmetrical developments may well balance—with no net significance for neck pain. In a left-handed

Normal leg length   Shorter right leg

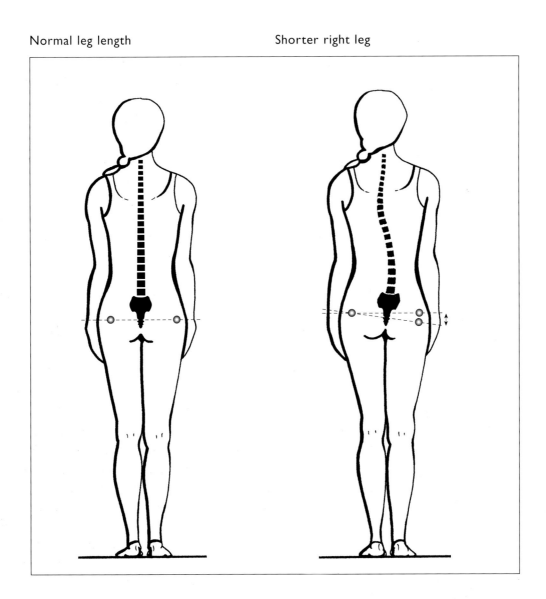

person, the effects may compound and cause neck pain through segmental nerve impingement, muscle tension, or other mechanisms. Other external factors such as the uneven muscular development caused by an asymmetric sport (golf, for example) may be cumulative or countervailing causes for similar reasons. Focusing on function is the best way to consider the problem, both diagnostically and curatively.

What is good posture?

Most people assume that the body is symmetrical because our faces look symmetrical, we have two hands, two legs, and so on. However, this is rarely true. Asymmetry is often visible just by looking at someone carefully. Similarly, the disposition of the internal organs is not symmetrical. The liver is located on the right hand side of your abdomen (the left from another's perspective), and the stomach on the left. The lungs are also of different sizes, with the heart nestling more inside the left one.

Good posture is not a form imposed on our own structure, as an externally-applied ideal. Some bodywork schools attempt to impose an ideal of posture by creating good postural

Schematic of good posture

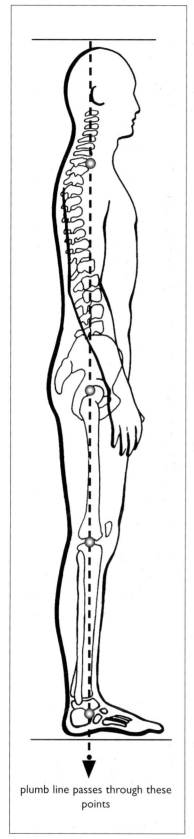

plumb line passes through these points

habits. In this approach, the individual consciously imposes certain ways of moving or holding the body. The approach relies on repeating these self-instructions until they become one's own ways of moving and holding the body.

However, the imposition of mental models alone is generally not a very efficient way to alter the basic structure and function of one's body. Continual imposition of these models can result in a somewhat mechanical or 'robotic' way of moving that works against the spontaneity of good movement. Until the models themselves have 'become' you, you tend to forget the ideal form when you are distracted or fatigued. Good posture should be effortless and involuntary—most babies and animals have perfect posture. The path to gracefulness and ease of movement does not need additional constraints. This is not to deny that the many hours of repetition of movements done by dancers and gymnasts (not to mention yoga teachers and the like) help to make them graceful in ordinary life. But unless you have these goals foremost in your life, it is inefficient to use these approaches to gain ease of movement and good posture.

A better approach for most people is to apply certain kinds of stress to the body so that the body itself changes. Sufficient change yields good posture and graceful movement. The spin-offs are a reduction in pain and a feeling of physical freedom. In contrast to animals and babies, adults can pursue these goals efficiently, by analysing their own form and applying corrective techniques. The most significant differences between adults and babies or animals are awareness and knowledge, and these can be used to improve posture and ease of movement.

According to physiotherapists (Kendall *et al.*, 1971, p.19) good posture may be determined using a plumb line. If the body is viewed from the side, and if the weight of the plumb line is placed a little forward of one ankle bone (*malleolus*), the line attached to the weight will pass slightly forward of the axis of the knee joint and slightly behind the axis of the hip joint. The line will be parallel with a number of lumbar vertebrae, run through the shoulder joint, and align with the back of the ear. Examine the illustration. From the side the body is not by any means straight. The curves of the spine are clear. In this plane (the sagittal plane) the shape of the spine can be seen as the solution to a number of conflicting needs—to absorb shock (especially from running or walking), to protect the spinal cord, and *to use the minimum amount of energy to maintain its shape*. This last consideration has major implications for the concerns of this book.

Notice that there is no symmetry in this plane. The front half (that section forward of the line) bears no relation in terms of shape to the back half. However, if a person with good posture is standing in a relaxed fashion, about half of the body's weight will be on either side of this line. The centre of gravity in the average person is slightly in front of the first or second sacral segment (recall that the sacrum is the lowest, fused part of the spine). This suggests that the centre of gravity roughly coincides with the hip joint.

In contrast, the symmetry of the body is clear from behind—a right and a left half. Good posture is regarded as having the ankles in a stable configuration, neither rolling in nor out. The Achilles tendon should be straight from the heel to the calf muscle. The legs should appear straight, with the hips level. The spine should be straight, with the shoulders level and the head held above the spine and in line with it.

Ideal posture is that shape the body adopts as its 'minimum-energy configuration'—the shape that requires the minimum amount of energy to support. Try this little experiment. Stand up and place the back of one hand horizontally across the small of your back. Alter the inclination of the body very slightly forwards or backwards, until you find a point where the large muscles running up both sides of the spine are completely relaxed. These muscles are relaxed even though you are standing up and supporting the body's weight. Ligaments, tendons, and joints are providing the support. Now lean forwards from this position. Immediately, these long muscles tighten considerably—even though the weight of the body has not changed. By leaning forward though, the configuration of the body did change, and hence the muscles were required to do extra work. From this example, you can see that if your posture is inefficient by even a small amount, you must do a considerable amount of extra work to support your body.

Assuming this idea of minimum-energy configuration is correct, your structure (the alignment of the body) or your available range of movement may not permit you to realise this form. Your minimum-energy shape may in fact require quite an effort. To return to the theme of an earlier paragraph, there is not much point in trying to impose an ideal form on a less than ideal structure. Optimal results are gained by working at the structural level, working slowly to change the shape of the spine and its support mechanisms.

Consider the body from the side view in more detail. With respect to neck pain, one needs to assess whether the curve of the thoracic spine is excessive. Recall the simple experiment. Although everyone's body is unique, if your head is carried sufficiently far in front of the shoulders, all the neck muscles involved in extension (that is, the muscles which bring the head backwards) will be contracted whenever you are in the normal vertical load-bearing position—even when you are sitting down. The main thing to look for is whether the curve of the thoracic spine is causing you to hold the head *in front* of that ideal posited position. If this is so, various muscles are doing work that is unnecessary in a better-balanced person, simply to hold your head level.

A similar analysis applies to the shape of the lumbar spine. Although excessive lumbar curve (lumbar *lordosis*, or 'sway' back) is often cited as a cause of low back pain, this explanation may be a little simplistic. Sometimes, someone with well-developed buttocks can give the impression of sway back to a casual inspection that mistakes the curve of the buttocks for the course of the spine. The shape of the whole spine needs to be considered. For example, many

Simple model of possible effects of leg-length difference

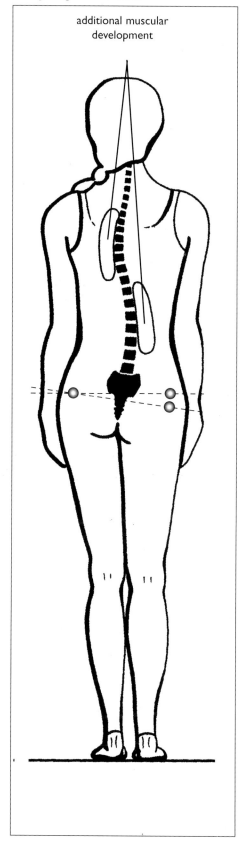

additional muscular development

a dancer or gymnast gives the impression of having a sway back for the reason just given, but has a thoracic spine with an ideal gentle curve, and shoulders that sit squarely, and a head carried perfectly. This is not a true sway back. Such athletes usually have very powerful abdominal muscles (which play an important support role) so that even if (technically speaking) one of them *does* have a sway back, it may be well compensated and hence not maladaptive.

In some people, very tight lower back muscles can prevent the spine's normal reverse curve from straightening, let alone allowing it to bend forward. This, too, can give the impression of a sway back. Some people also have a more pronounced curve in the lumbar spine, but without any dysfunctionality, and with great mobility. To label such form as a sway back serves little purpose. Finally, just because there is no symmetry between the front and back halves of the body, the determination and assessment of 'normal' remains problematic.

When one looks at the body from behind, asymmetry may be seen relatively easily. Perhaps of most importance with respect to neck and back pain is the height of the hips. If one leg is anatomically shorter than the other, the hip bone will be carried lower on that side. This has implications for the shape of the whole spine. Leaving aside questions of the effects of right–left arm dominance for a moment, if the right leg is actually shorter than the left, then the three normal curves of the spine in the plane we have been considering will be reproduced subtly in the plane running through both shoulders. The left shoulder will then be carried on the outside of a gently right-curving thoracic spine, as shown in the illustration.

To the untrained eye, a difference in shoulder height may be difficult to see. It is often easier to appreciate by considering whether the fingers of one hand reach further down one leg than the other, assuming that the arms are the same length. Alternatively, if looking at the body from behind, the course of the spine may be more easily seen by inclining the body forward from the hips, as in the experiment mentioned above (the tightened muscles highlight the shape of the spine, especially if lit from the side).

Various factors may mask the differences mentioned. One arm may be longer than the other. You can check this by lying down with the shoulders resting on the floor and extending the arms up from the chest, with the fingers brought together over the centre of the chest. Another person can check this for you. As mentioned, right or left arm dominance can mask other adaptations. In the example of a short right leg producing an elevated left shoulder, the elevation deriving from the leg-length difference will tend to be increased in a left-handed person due to the greater development of the shoulder and neck muscles on the left side. In contrast, a right-handed person may show perfectly level shoulders, even with the shorter right leg. Here, one adaptation is balanced with another so that there is no easily visible difference. Despite appearing symmetrical to the casual observer, such a person may still suffer from neck or back pain from the asymmetrical distribution of forces around the lower back and neck due to the leg-length inequality. Visual inspection cannot be guaranteed to reveal all that one needs to know to solve problems.

To the notion of *structural* asymmetry needs to be added the idea (another layer in effect) of *functional* symmetry—a comparison of symmetry of function, derived from a consideration of both structural and functional aspects. Functional means the observable function that derives not only from the levers of the body (the skeleton) but also the muscles, ligaments, tendons, and nerves. All of these are overlaid with acquired patterns of movement, mental attitude and so on—all the possible factors that contribute to the way the body functions at any given time.

Consider, for example, a 'sweep' rower. In this sport, the body's power is transmitted to the oar through an arc of considerable size. See the illustration. The arm on the outside of this arc travels further (as does its shoulder). In the case of a rower sitting on the left-hand side of the boat, all the muscles of the right-hand side of the spine contract through a wider arc. A significant component of rotation is thus added to the fundamental extension movement of rowing. Over time, if the athlete always rows on the same side of the boat, the muscles of the back develop unevenly. This means that even a rower who is perfectly balanced (structurally speaking) will acquire (and display) uneven function, both in terms of flexibility and strength. This alone can contribute significantly to back pain. Even if you are not a competitive athlete, similar movements can affect you. For example, if you play golf or tennis, or always turn your head strongly each day only in the one direction (which side do you look over as you back the car out of the garage each day?), you are likely to develop similar asymmetry.

Testing functional flexibility does not require a complex set of tests to be administered by an expert. It merely refers to a selection of the stretching exercises covered in chapter one. The key functions to be tested for are (with respect to back pain) right and left lateral flexion and right and left rotation of the spine. Because of the lack of symmetry between the front and back halves of the body, no absolute standards can be suggested for comparisons of flexion and extension in the individual case. However, each half of the body should be the same or very similar, so regardless of your flexibility in absolute terms, the flexibility of each half of the trunk (in both the movements mentioned), and each arm and leg should ideally be the same.

There is no necessary relation between flexion and extension. A person who is unusually flexible in extension may be anywhere between flexible and stiff in flexion. Beyond stating that you should improve your flexibility within the limits of your strength, it is impossible to specify desirable limits for these functions. The spine is far more flexible bending backwards than forwards (apart from its structure, the ribs obstruct flexion of the thoracic spine, and the chest blocks forward movement of the chin, thus limiting flexion of the cervical spine).

Schematic of rowing

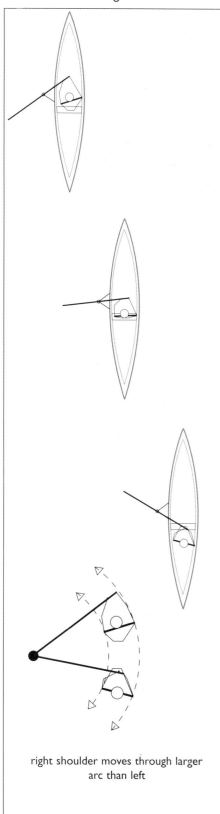

right shoulder moves through larger
arc than left

Maximally-flexible individuals can exhibit up to 110 degrees of flexion and up to 140 degrees of extension (Kapandji, 1974, vol. III, p. 44). Note that these figures are estimated with respect to the plane of the bite, and thus include the possible movements of the entire spine.

If anything, Kapandji underestimated the possible degree of freedom of the lumbar spine in extension (he gives 35 degrees). His illustration of a yoga pose on the same page supports this objection. In any case, the trained individual has considerable freedom of movement available. Within limits, improving the range of movement of the individual parts of the spine (providing there is sufficient strength to support the movement) will make the body feel looser and more relaxed. It will also help the body to settle into a form that is closer to the minimum-energy configuration.

When we consider the spine from behind, we can be more certain in our prescriptions. In general, right and left lateral flexion should be the same, because the structures are symmetrical. Right and left rotation, while involving structures from the anterior–posterior plane that we admitted have no necessary symmetry, also involve the symmetrical plane in each rotational range. Because the same halves of each structure (front to back) are involved in rotation on each side, these movements should also be symmetrical. However, usually they are not. The degree of total movement in this plane may suggest additional checking of the degree of freedom of the hip flexors and extensors. For example, if you cannot lie face-up and press the lower back flat onto the floor with the legs held straight, it is likely that your hip flexors are too tight. This will contribute to certain kinds of back pain.

Looking at the region of the upper back and neck, we expect to see a balanced structure. Things to look for include the way the head is carried on the neck, how the neck is carried on the shoulders, and the elevation of respective shoulders. Consider whether the thoracic spine is straight. As with the lumbar spine, a slight forward inclination of the upper body can reveal a lateral curve, particularly if lit from the side. Look at how the arms are carried. Is one arm rotated more inwardly than the other? This may indicate that the front shoulder muscle or the biceps muscle on this side is tighter than on the other. If there is no problem with the arm or shoulder, this difference is merely something to keep an eye on. If there is a problem, these muscles should be looked at first.

The main exercises to test your functional flexibility are (in order of importance) right and left lateral flexion of the spine (treat the neck as part of the spine), and right and left rotation of the whole spine. The neck and the lower back may be tested separately. Follow this by testing hip flexibility (hip flexion) and the hamstring group. Then test hip extension. If this appears markedly deficient, also test quadriceps flexibility, which is often correlated with hip extension. If lateral flexion or rotation of the neck is found to be impaired, test shoulder flexibility, especially the movements which stretch the front shoulder muscles and the long head of the biceps muscle. Do not test extension movements of the spine (including the neck) if there is any acute pain, because extension movements tend to aggravate this condition.

The keys to good posture are ease and efficiency. First and foremost, your posture needs to be pain-free and feel 'easy', effortless, and graceful. Secondly, the form of the body at any time needs to be efficient, or require a minimum of effort to support. Looking at this another way, good posture also allows the strength of the body to be used easily. Good posture allows the widest distribution of forces and hence enables the body in the most general sense. For this reason, there is not only one kind of good posture. Different proportions and different personal histories make an absolute or universal determination of good posture impossible. Your task is to work on your own body to make it work as well as it can and to define your own best posture. Working with your body in the ways described will facilitate the unconscious acquisition of this most important attribute.

For practitioners

My observations, drawn from years of working with sufferers of neck and back pain and years of working with athletes, are set out below and may be of assistance to practitioners. The following section describes the tests used to determine leg-length difference. If you are not a practitioner, you may do these tests with another person if you wish, or you can skip this section and proceed directly to the following chapter.

In the conventional lying face-up approach to testing leg length, the practitioner holds the patient's heels just off the bench, and applies an equal, gentle pull to both legs. The comparison is made by examining the heels. If one is closer to the practitioner, it is judged to be the longer leg. The problem with this test is that other factors may mask the difference completely, or even submerge it. In the extreme case the leg appearing as the longer one in this test may

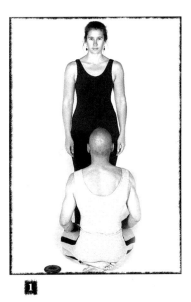

1

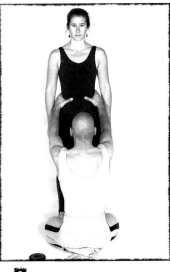

2

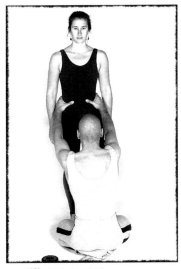

3 Left hip higher

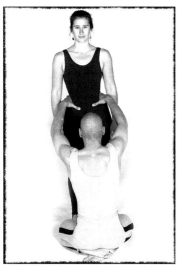

4 Right hip higher

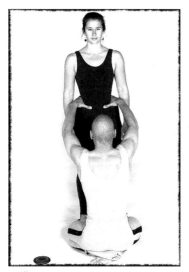

5 Centre position

actually be shorter than its partner. For example, if the patient has occasioned trauma to *quadratus lumborum*, the oblique group of muscles, or the deep muscles of the lumbar spine, their contraction alone (in response to the trauma) will draw the hip on that side towards the ribs when the body is relaxed, or supported. This contraction can give the impression of the leg on the side of the injury being the shorter one, and another test described below reveals the opposite. Leg-length testing must be done in the standing position, because in the lying position, muscular contractions can pull the pelvis one way or another. It may be objected that the contracted muscles will disturb the alignment of the pelvis. However, in the standing position with the body's weight firmly over both feet, the body itself will be distorted—that is, the body alone will be drawn to the side of the injury. As the practitioner's concern is with the height of the hips, this distortion can be ignored for the purpose of determining leg length.

In the next series of photographs, Jennifer is the patient. Kneeling in front of the patient, place your hands on both sides of the patient's waist. Observe, and gently move the hips from one side to the other (a centimetre or two) and ask the patient to tell you when both feet feel as though they have the same amount of weight on them. At the same time, you are feeling the muscles on each side of the waist contract in turn as you move the hips in either direction, and this will also help you locate the mid-point. This central position (with respect to a mark on the wall, say) becomes the reference. Repeat if necessary without looking at the reference mark. Check the patient's position with respect to the reference mark when tension in the waist muscles feels balanced. Again ask the patient if she feels that her weight is being borne equally by both feet.

Now place the base of both index fingers at the highest point of the iliac crests, with the palms of your hands level with the floor (see photographs). We assume that if the height of the crests is unequal, the difference is due to a leg-length difference. This may be confirmed by marking the position of the *greater trochanter* (the palpable knob of the thigh bone just below the hip joint) and viewing the marks from in front of the patient. Any difference in the height of the iliac crests is probably due to an actual leg-length difference. Of course, it is possible that a patient may have *ilia* of different heights or an uneven location of the hip joint with respect to the iliac crest, but at the scale of leg-length difference we are considering (a centimetre) these differences usually will not be significant. If you do suspect this sort of anomaly, you may determine the location of the greater trochanter by checking the location of the axis of the hip joint and the iliac crests on both sides.

In some patients, leg-length difference may be difficult to detect, either because of the patient's shape or physical condition, or because the difference is small. To magnify the difference (and to involve the patient further) I use a piece of wood about a centimetre thick, placed alternately under one foot then the other. Wood is a desirable material for this test because it assumes room temperature. Ask the patient to place his or her weight evenly over both feet once more. When the piece of wood is under the *longer* leg, the difference in height of the hips is easily seen. Under the shorter leg, the hips seem level. This simple test can be confirmed by asking the patient to face away from you and repeating the test for confirmation. You can also ask the patient to lean forward from the hips a few centimetres with the skin and muscles of the lumbar region in view. This reveals the shape of the spine clearly, and placing the piece of wood will confirm the location of the shortness. For confirming evidence, ask to see a worn pair of shoes. Generally, although not always, the sole of the shoe of the shorter leg is the more worn.

Few studies have examined the prevalence of leg-length inequality in the general population. The authors of a review of six studies concluded that 'about 7% (range 4–8%) of the adult population with no history of low back pain have lower limb inequality of 1 cm or more' (Giles and Taylor, 1985). Assuming that leg-length difference plays a causal role in back pain (and perhaps neck pain too), it would be expected that the proportion of people suffering neck or back pain who display this difference would be greater than in the general population.

In my clinic, about 75% of patients with chronic back pain have a significant difference in leg length. The difference is significant if determinable by the test mentioned—if there is no apparent difference, it may be that there is no difference or that the difference is one which the body can cope with without too much problem. This proportion is much higher than that reported in other studies (for example, Giles and Taylor, 1985, who state 18.3% and Rock, 1988, who states 10.9%). Part of the apparent discrepancy in these figures is due to the nine millimetre threshold chosen in the studies. For example, Rock's study found that a further 38.5% of the chronic sufferers had a leg length difference of between five and nine millimetres. Differences as small as 4 or 5 millimetres may be significant in small patients. Another explanation for the much higher percentage of patients displaying leg-length inequality in my clinic may be that I am seeing a proportion of patients who have not responded to other approaches, and in whom leg length difference is a causal factor.

Let us assume that you have found a leg-length difference and you have confirmed it by retesting from behind. Let us say that the difference seems to be a centimetre. How much correction should be used? Before considering a specific amount, let us review the argument. My approach is partly based on the claim that a lateral curvature of the spine induced by a leg-length difference can cause back pain, probably through the uneven work done by the muscles of the laterally-curved spine. In many patients, this asymmetry is compensated by additional development of the muscles stabilising the pelvis in the transverse plane *opposite* the shorter leg (lumbar spine) and also on the side of the shorter leg (thoracic spine). However, this compensation provides two loci for pain, through two mechanisms. One is nerve impingement, and the other is simple muscular soreness brought about by particular muscles on one side of the spine having to do more work than on the other. This produces more development in the affected muscles, but the muscles are shorter (normal state more contracted) and they are closer to the fatigued state than the opposite side's weaker, though more relaxed, counterparts. This may explain in part the oft-reported tendency for episodes of back pain to follow periods of stress or fatigue—that is, the affected muscles reach their limit for doing work before the others. However, these predictions of muscular development are not always borne out in practice, and (despite any predictive models to the contrary) one must deal with each patient *as he or she present themselves to you*. Other causes may confound the expectations I have outlined here. In such cases, deal with the functional or structural asymmetry you find.

Another related likely cause is the nerve impingement mechanism mentioned above. That is, in daily life the intervertebral foramina are narrower on the side of the longer leg, because the spine is tilted in this direction to distribute its load as evenly as possible and to achieve balance in all of life's activities. This adaptation is especially significant in upright load-bearing positions, and thus more likely to be causal in people who spend their life on their feet, or whose sport places similar demands on the skeleton.

It will be clear from the discussion so far that the greater the leg-length difference, the greater its significance as a possible causal factor, even if other possible causes are present. A minor difference is unlikely to be significant, because it is within the body's capacity to adapt *without negative consequences*. Accordingly, the last millimetres of any difference are more significant (with respect to the problem) than the first millimetres. Addressing the extreme part of the difference is thus more likely to yield positive benefits than addressing a difference which is closer to the balanced position. If one patient has a leg-length difference of 10 millimetres and another has a difference of 3 millimetres, inserting a lift of 3 millimetres into the shoe of the shorter leg will yield far more dramatic results in the patient with the larger difference. The reason is that back pain, like any other, is a phenomenon with a threshold. If stimulation is below the threshold, pain is not experienced, even though the cause of the stimulation may be present. The 3 millimetre insert causes the same change in angle of the pelvis with respect to the theoretical transverse plane in both cases (let us say a few degrees). However, the change is of greater significance in the patient with the larger leg-length difference because the lateral curvature of this patient's spine is closer to the threshold where capacity for work or impingement is reached.

For these reasons, an insert of between 3 and 6 millimetres should be used in most cases. A greater thickness is not recommended for three reasons. Assuming that the patient has adapted during life to this structural difference (even if the adaptation is incomplete or only partially effective), correcting the whole difference will render these adaptations maladaptive, and hence likely to cause other problems. The second reason is a practical one. Most shoe styles will accept an insert of this thickness without the discomfort of the heel not being securely held in the shoe. The third reason is one of economy. If a small correction yields the desired result, it is to be preferred. It is a basic tenet of physical medicine to use the smallest stimulation of the body's adaptive mechanisms which will serve the desired purpose, and have the least risk of undesirable side effects.

In cases where there is back pain but no discernible leg-length difference, consider *function*—the 'global' properties of the person, such as the ability to flex at the hip, or the capacity to rotate at the waist. The term global refers to those macro-scale properties of the whole person

175

that arise through the properties of a number of smaller parts—bones, nerves, ligaments, muscles and so on. Any global property cannot be directly traced to any single sub-system but arises from the particular arrangement of these systems, together with their individual properties.

As discussed above, from the structure of the skeleton, we infer that certain functions will be symmetrical—right–left lateral flexion of any part of the spine, and right–left rotation—simply because of the symmetry of the skeletal structure in the planes concerned. In cases of back pain where no significant leg-length difference can been detected (and hence no significant skeletal asymmetry), functional symmetry should be examined to determine if other long-term influences may be present.

Two major symmetries need to be considered, and two comparisons be made, to gain an understanding of the significant functions. These are right–left lateral flexion (of the relevant part of the spine—that is, lower back, middle back, or neck), and right–left rotation of the same structures. The only equipment needed is a massage table or a firm mat on the floor. Right-left lateral flexion needs to be tested on the floor, as the floor can be used to stabilise the pelvis laterally. The test position is the same as in exercise 18, *C–R and partner version of legs apart*. The present section refers to the partner-assisted lateral exercise for lateral flexion over one leg. Refer to these photographs now. Ask the patient to sit on the floor with legs as far apart as comfortable, and to turn to one side so that the shoulders are in line with one leg. Then ask the patient to lean to one side. If the pain of the original complaint is unilateral, ask the patient to lean carefully *away* from the painful area for the first stretch. Estimates of tightness or inflexibility, or elicitation of pain will necessarily involve the patient. We are not seeking an objective measure or comparison of right–left symmetry so much as a combination of your observations together with the patient's reported sensations.

At least two outcomes are possible. When the patient leans away from the painful area, he or she may say that, on returning to the starting position, the pain is diminished. This indicates that the source of the pain is likely to be muscular. If, on leaning to the painful side the patient complains of an intensified pain or of referred pain in the leg or elsewhere, this indicates that segmental nerve impingement may be the likely cause. Note that, although the starting position of the test has the shoulders in line with one leg, you may need to ask the patient to roll the top shoulder inwards to duplicate the pain. Do this especially if you suspect that the deep lumbar muscles are responsible, because the small additional flexion induced involves these additional muscles. Tightness in the hamstring muscles holds the pelvis in position, and this is why it is recommended that the testing be done on the floor with the legs outstretched. The main muscle group being stretched in the test is *quadratus lumborum*, with the oblique groups also being affected. The obliques are not the source of back pain for most patients, so this effect may safely be ignored.

When a patient is too inflexible in the hamstring group or the hip adductors to sit on the floor in the first position, it may be necessary to duplicate the test in the seated position. Here the body's weight is supported and the knees flexed. The accompanying photograph shows the chair version of this test. Usually, these alterations to the preferred position will still yield useful test results. In this test, the practitioner is looking for a comparison of right-left lateral flexion, how this makes the patient feel, and, sometimes importantly, what happens to the shape of the spine in the other plane to the one being examined. In some patients, the degree

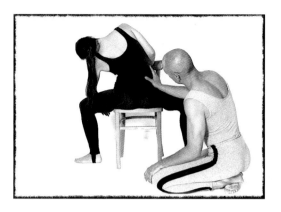

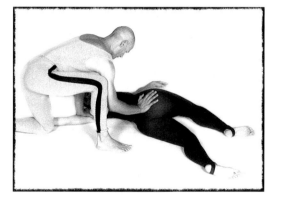

of freedom in comparisons of flexion may appear similar, but the patient needs to flex or extend the spine further when turning to one side. In addition to a visual comparison, the practitioner needs to ask the patient what effects are being experienced during the test.

The preferred test of lumbar rotation is performed in the lying position. Look at the photograph. The patient's knee is flexed to around 90 degrees, as is the hip. The patient's opposite shoulder is held onto the mat with firm pressure on the front of the shoulder. As the patient brings the leg to the test position, ensure that the hip resting on the mat slides underneath a similar amount (ask the patient to lift the hip up and back for you), so that when viewed from above, the patient's spine appears straight. This is essential to prevent hyperextension of the lumbar spine, which could confuse the results, or cause a confounding pain through pressure on the facet joints. Do not press on the knee of the bent leg when doing the test, but apply a small amount of pressure to the buttock of the bent leg, at the position indicated. This avoids any pinching in the hip joint itself.

If the patient has unequal adduction capacity in the hip joints, the knee may come closer to the floor on the looser hip's side if force is applied to the knee. This occurs through adduction, *not* through greater lumbar rotational capacity, and will confuse the test results. Estimate the distance of the test leg's knee from the mat, and then retest the other side. During both parts of the test, ask the patient to report any sensations. It is likely that a patient demonstrating reduced hip flexion on, say, the right side will demonstrate a similar tightness when taking the right leg down to the mat. This is even more likely if the patient's right leg is the longer one. These observations suggest shorter lower back muscles on the right side (commensurate with the model outlined above), and the combination of results suggests involvement of the *quadratus lumborum* muscle groups.

Although there is no front–back symmetry in the body, no tests for low back pain would be complete without a comparison of right–left hip flexion, right–left hamstring, and right–left hip extension. This is because these muscle groups can directly affect both the shape of the spine and positions of particular vertebrae with respect to one another. The results of these further tests will need to be interpreted in the light of the above tests, as discussed below.

Although it is commonly believed that tight hamstring muscles can cause back pain, the mechanism of this is not described. Kapandji notes that as the hamstrings contract, they flatten the lumbar curve (v. III, p.106), so their action militates against other muscles' actions that increase the curve—an increased curve often being cited as a possible cause of back pain. The reason hamstring muscles are correctly implicated in back pain is probably that, if they are particularly tight, much forward bending in normal life is achieved by flexion of the spine (flattening of the lumbar curve) rather than at the hip joint. Bending this way accentuates the shearing forces already present at the L5–S1 interface (the lumbosacral joint), increasing wear and tear, and predisposing the patient to disc injury at this level. Bending this way also requires the extensors of the spine to contract or lengthen under load which can cause fatigue or muscle spasm, especially if combined with rotation. These effects may occur even when the hamstring muscles are sufficiently loose to permit efficient movement, through poor movement patterns (that is, by bending forward from the lumbar spine rather than from the hips).

Remember that one hamstring muscle (*biceps femoris*) is attached to the femur for much of its length. Thus the hamstring group as a whole may test within normal limits, but the section of *biceps femoris* between the pelvis and the femur can still restrict flexion of the hip. This is because the normal hamstring test with the leg straight is completed somewhere between 50–90 degrees in the normally-flexible individual. If *biceps femoris* is limiting hip flexion, it will only be revealed by a hip joint test with knee flexed at around the 110–120 degrees point (with the floor as reference). The error occurs because it is common to think of the hamstring as a single muscle spanning both the hip joint and the knee, when in fact it is three separate muscles with different attachments and origins, and overlapping functions. The first photograph on the following page shows a test for *biceps femoris*.

Of perhaps more interest for the practitioner concerned with back pain is a *comparison* of hamstring tightness. The hamstring muscle of the shorter leg is usually the looser of the two (anteroposteriorally), as is the hip joint of the shorter leg in this plane. Test results may thus add weight to the determination of a short leg. Remember that chiropractors and doctors regard 8 or 9 millimetres as the threshold of significance. If you find that the tests mentioned show a pattern confirming what might be expected with a shorter leg and yet the difference in length you identified was not significant, you may wish to reconsider your first determination. In my view, any difference *may* be significant—the determination cannot be made by measurement of the legs alone. A difference in hamstring flexibility in a patient who is an athlete may be significant for other reasons. This is because of the unequal stresses produced around the sacrum during training and during the event itself. This seems particularly significant for distance runners.

The accompanying photograph shows the recommended test. The leg *must* be moved into the test position extremely carefully (that is, slowly and gently). This is especially important if sciatic pain from nerve impingement is suspected, because the nerve roots are pulled out from the foramina for up to 12 millimetres at the L5 level in the flexible person during the test. Incautious elevation of the leg can produce sufficient traction on the nerve to rupture

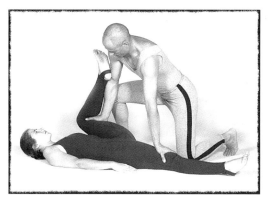

1

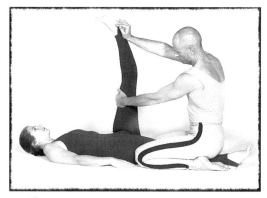

Test of hip flexion

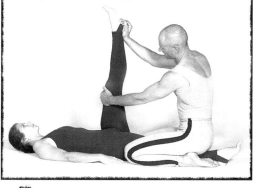

2

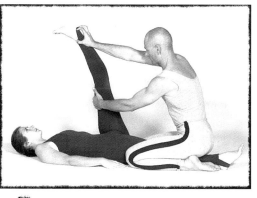

3

some of the involved axons (nerve fibres) which may result in paralysis (Kapandji, 1974, vol. III, p.126).

Sit over the non-test leg as shown. Lean back, hold the test leg at the heel, and raise the leg *slowly and gently*. As you do this, place a restraining hand on the thigh above the knee (between the knee and the hip), to keep the leg straight. Pain felt anywhere along the leg or in the back elicited in any part of the range of movement between horizontal and 45 degrees is regarded as a *positive Lasègue's sign*, indicative of nerve root involvement. Note that Kapandji states up to 60 degrees, but my clinical experience suggests that for many normal individuals who simply have tight hamstrings, 45 degrees is a more useful figure. If the leg goes past the 60 degrees point, there is little chance of sciatic nerve involvement as maximum tension in the nerve is reached at this position, and does not increase as the leg is lifted further (Kapandji, 1974, vol. III, p. 126).

Pain felt at the back of the leg between the buttock and the area just below the back of the knee may be a *false* positive sign. To distinguish between tight hamstrings and nerve involvement, at the point where pain is first felt, ask the patient exactly where the pain is. To confirm, ask the patient to press the leg down to the floor gently for a few seconds while you maintain the leg's position. Wait for a breath in and as the patient breathes out, very gently elevate the leg. If the pain was caused by tight hamstrings, the leg will go past the initial point to a new stretch position. If nerve root involvement is present it will not. These tests *must* be done extremely carefully. Hoppenfeld suggests dorsiflexing the patient's ankle (moving the ball of foot towards knee) at the point pain is first felt. If referred pain is not experienced, the test pain is probably due to tight hamstrings (Hoppenfeld, 1976, p.256). My experience suggests that adding this stretch is quite likely to increase the pain felt all the way along the back of the leg. This is often due to a tight *gastrocnemius* (calf) muscle.

The functional relationship between the respective strengths and flexibilities of *iliopsoas* and *quadratus lumborum* is not adequately researched in my view. In addition to their role in shaping the lumbar curve, these muscles play a critical role in the rotational stability of lumbar vertebrae. *Iliopsoas* has fibres that attach to the anterior processes of each lumbar vertebra. *Quadratus lumborum*'s fibres attach to the posterior processes of the lumbar vertebrae, as well as having fine fibres spanning the distance between the iliac crest and the last rib. Ideally, the forces generated by these muscles should balance, both at the level of the individual vertebra as well as the lumbar curve as a whole. Alternatively, if these forces occur sequentially (as with any movement), the forces should balance *over time*. Balance thus needs to be considered in dynamic terms in addition to what static tests may reveal. The forces produced by the energetic movements of sport or energetic exercise are far greater than those typically produced in static situations. For a fuller causal picture, the practitioner needs to analyse the particular demands a patient places on his or her body.

Vertebral stability can be upset reasonably easily. It is not unusual to find that a weakness or tightness in a single set of fibres is sufficient to rotate one vertebra with respect to its neighbours. Considering both muscle groups, it is not at all unusual to find excessive lumbar lordosis caused by shortness of the *iliopsoas* group (through the pull on the anterior surfaces of the transverse processes), and that the resulting anterior tilt of the pelvis is accompanied by shortness of both *quadratus lumborum* and the extensors of the spine. Back pain is often blamed on weakness in the abdominal muscles (whose contractions tend to flatten the lumbar curve). However, tight *iliopsoas* can easily overwhelm even strong abdominal muscles, due to their relative strengths and the additional extension *iliopsoas* causes to the spine during walking and other normal movement. This is partly due to the length of the legs, which are levers of great length that can easily exert enough force on *iliopsoas* to affect the lumbar curve. Tests show that only very rarely are the abdominal muscles strong enough to stretch *iliopsoas*. Remember that the conventional 'sit-up' exercise strengthens *iliopsoas* more than the abdominal groups. The common prescription of these exercises to strengthen the abdominals usually worsens the initial imbalance—that is, *iliopsoas* becomes even stronger than the abdominals through this activity.

During walking and running, all the leg muscles are used to move the body over the foot. As the leg passes the midline of the body, *iliopsoas* pulls the lumbar curve into further extension or rotates the pelvis in the transverse plane, following the leg if there is insufficient flexibility. In the muscularly-balanced and sufficiently-flexible person, even the much more exaggerated action of running does not appreciably change the lumbar curve, as slow-motion photography has shown. Although these effects are likely to be exacerbated by a leg-length difference, they can be present even when the legs are of identical lengths. A muscular imbalance can arise through use patterns, injury, or the like. For this reason any functional imbalance must be treated if found—even in the absence of structural differences.

There is one factor that complicates this analysis. Most anatomists agree that the lumbar curves were an adaptation facilitating the transition from four legs to two in our distant past. In the 'on all fours' position (on the hands and knees) the anterior ligaments of the hip (*iliofemoral, pubofemoral* and *ischiofemoral*) are relaxed, and run roughly coincident with the neck of the femur, similar to quadrupedal mammals. In humans standing in the normal erect posture, these ligaments are under moderate tension. This skeletal position would correspond to strong extension of the hip joint in quadrupedal mammals. Any movement of the leg back from the midline from the erect position *strongly* tightens these ligaments, which are by this stage wound around the neck of the femur. These ligaments are considerably less extensible

As leg extends, hip joint ligaments tighten around neck of femur

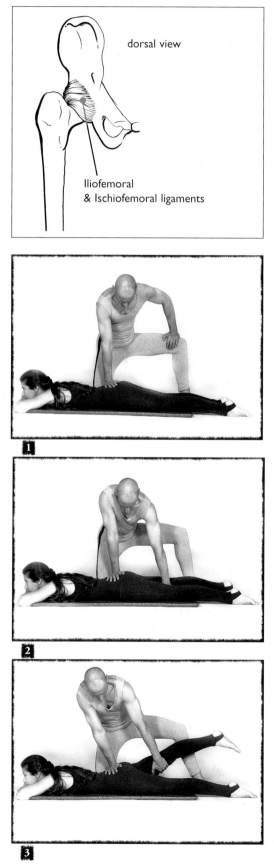

dorsal view

Iliofemoral
& Ischiofemoral ligaments

1

2

3

than the *iliopsoas* group of muscles discussed above. Therefore, it is essential to determine which of these structures is limiting the normal degree of required extension, of the sort necessary for walking or running. Two tests are offered.

Look at the photograph. The patient is lying face-down. Place your hand on the sacrum. Ensure that your weight is bearing on the patient vertically, and that you are in the stable position shown. Reach between the patient's legs and slide the fingers around the leg above the knee. Notice that both arms are straight so that the applied load derives from moving your whole body's weight around the fulcrum, the hand on the sacrum. While holding the leg, lean towards the patient's head, lifting the leg cautiously into a stretch position. Ask the patient to report any pain. Stop either at the point pain is elicited, or when a limit to the movement is felt. Normal flexibility is about 20 degrees *without* any hyperextension of the lumbar curve (your hand holding the sacrum must prevent any additional tilting of the pelvis). To determine whether the ligaments or *iliopsoas* are limiting, ask the patient to press the test leg back to the floor gently for a few seconds while you maintain the leg's position. Wait a few seconds and retest. If the leg moves further backwards, *iliopsoas* is likely to be the limiting structure, because the ligaments do not respond to the C–R approach.

For the second test, refer for a moment to exercise 20, *iliopsoas* (salute to the sun), *with partner; C–R*. The position described for a partner-assisted version of this movement is the best test position. With most patients, the practitioner will be able to see the difference in movement of the leg with respect to the body. With some, the practitioner will be required to ask for the patient's impressions of tightness or pain.

If excessive tightness in the hip flexors is found, the practitioner should additionally test *quadriceps*. The side of the tighter hip flexor will usually test tighter for *quadriceps* too. The test for *quadriceps* is the standard test performed in the lying face-down position, wherein each foot in turn is gently brought back to the buttocks for comparison (not shown). In any instance of unequal tightness, select the appropriate partner exercise from exercise 24, *quadriceps (standing; lying; C–R)*. Once or twice-weekly sessions to loosen the muscles involved should yield results within a couple of weeks.

One further cause of sciatica needs consideration. In about one fifth of the population, the perineal branch of the sciatic nerve pierces *piriformis*, one of the external hip rotators (Travell & Simons, 1992, vol. II, p. 186 ff.) rather than passing inferior to it. If this muscle is in spasm, enough clamping force can be produced on this branch of the sciatic nerve to cause pain in the muscles behind the hip joint and down the back of the leg. If such a patient has the kind of disc pathology that recent research has shown to exist in approximately two thirds of patients without back pain (Jensen *et al.*, 1994; these results were replicated with almost identical results in a recent study of the cervical spine), a diagnosis of nerve-impingement induced sciatica may be made without there being any causal relationship between pathology and symptom. None of the standard tests will identify *piriformis* as the cause of this kind of sciatica. The straight leg-lifting test will yield results consistent with disc-induced impingement, as *piriformis* in these patients will not permit the gliding of the sciatic nerve required by the test.

Practitioners confronted by patients suffering this excruciating pain may use exercise 9 (with C–R) as a test to identify the possibility of what we may call '*piriformis*-induced sciatica'. Should this test reproduce the hip pain aspect of the symptoms, I suggest that a suitably gentle form of exercise 36 be next tried, with the C–R component. In elderly patients, exercise 9 is sufficiently strong; in any case, some patients will not have sufficient flexibility to get into the starting position of exercise 36. I have found that about a third of the patients with sciatica I have seen in the last year responded favourably to a combination of these two exercises only. Exercises 27 and 28, and later 29, and 7 may be added as the patient progresses.

Exercise combinations for neck; upper, middle, and low back pain

For patients with neck pain, I recommend exercise 10 to start, followed by 11, 14, 13, and 15. The extension movement of exercise 11 may be omitted if painful, and the more gentle exercise 12 substituted when appropriate. Exercise 40 may be added when the pain has subsided.

In the general low back pain patients, the most successful minimum combination of exercises are exercises 3, 7 and the appropriate parts of 17 and 18 (or 4, 20 and 18 if a partner is available). If successful, additional exercises are 1 and 2, 21, a suitable version of 27, 28, and later 29. Usually I recommend that the routine be finished with a final iteration of exercise 3. When pain subsides, the extension movements covered in exercises 22, 23 and 24 may be added, but always to be followed by a back flexion movement. When the patient feels ready, strengthening exercise may be tried: exercise 38 to begin, and 37 a couple of weeks later.

For middle-back pain, I suggest exercises 1, 3, 5, 6, and both versions of 8. For upper back pain, exercise 11 may be added, and 35 when appropriate.

One year later

In this brief addendum to the *For practitioners* section, I wish to present further information resulting from the year's intensive work in the clinic following the release of the first edition of the book. As I noted in the *Afterword,* many readers wrote to me with suggestions, and some of these ideas are presented below.

My position with respect to the significance of the short-leg syndrome and its relation to both neck and back pain has been strengthened. Towards the end of last year, a colleague showed me his copy of the excellent book *Myofascial Pain and Dysfunction: The Trigger Point Manual* by Travell and Simons. Their chapter on 'Perpetuating Factors' (Travell & Simons, 1983, Vol. 1, pp. 103-164) is thorough, and I recommend it to all practitioners. Their survey and analysis of the literature and their vast clinical experience is a model of scholarship. Their findings with respect to the short-leg syndrome agree with the position taken in the first edition of this book, and provide a wealth of experimental and clinical evidence in support. Their analysis expands on mine in some respects, and it is to these points I wish to turn.

In addition to claiming that leg-length inequality is a major determinant of pain both in the back and the neck, they draw attention to a further sub-class of the problem, the 'small hemipelvis' (*ibid.,* p. 177 ff.) which may or may not be associated with a short leg. They recommend a test similar to the one I described earlier in this chapter, performed with the patient seated on a firm surface with the back and buttocks visible (see photograph p. 177). Examine the curve of the spine, and height of hips while the patient sits upright, before doing the recommended test. I suggest that this test be done if: i) the standing test indicates disparate iliac crest heights, yet the visible course of the spine appears straight, or   ii) levelling the iliac crests with a test correction in the clinic causes the spine to curve laterally, or iii) the patient complains of recurring back pain mainly while sitting (here, the patient may present a straight spine in the standing test, but will demonstrate an induced scoliosis when seated). Their recommendation for correction in patients of this kind is a support for the smaller half of the pelvis to be used when seated. Such patients may or may not require a leg-length correction. One additional source of structural misalignment which may ramify to an apparent leg-length inequality is when the sacrum is tilted in relation to the pelvis. This condition should be visible on an anteroposterior radiograph, and is able to be corrected by manipulation. In such cases, I recommend an analysis of the patient's structure and function as described earlier in this chapter, to try to determine the nature of the cause of this particular 'adaptation', presuming that trauma is not the cause.

Choice of bed

The recommendation is commonly made that a firm bed is the best kind for people with neck or back problems. My view is that this recommendation needs to be considered in relation to both your shape and your body weight. A firm *base* is desirable in any case, but one reader noted that a sagging base provided some relief for his back pain, largely caused by an excessive lumbar lordosis. I believe that one needs to choose a mattress or other support that deforms sufficiently to permit the buttocks to rest far enough below the surface of the rest of the bed that the lumbar spine feels comfortable. Accordingly, if you are a light person, you will find a too-firm mattress uncomfortable. If you have well-developed (prominent) buttocks, you too may need a softer mattress than is usually recommended. However, these remarks will need to be modified if you are relatively heavy. Overall, I think that the body needs to be supported in such a way as to allow the spine to be held in its most comfortable position. You will need to consider also the shape of the spine while lying on your side: ideally, in this position the spine should be as close to straight as possible. This means that a woman with wider hips might need a softer mattress than a man of similar weight, but with broader shoulders and narrower hips. A compromise in firmness that permits the best-possible face-up and lying-side positions is desirable.

As far as neck pain is concerned, my experience is that you need a pillow that is sufficiently firm and thick when compressed by the weight of the head to hold the head as close to the neutral position as possible *in the side lying position.* I suggest that no pillow be used when lying face-up. If you go to sleep in the lying face-up position, you may care to try to go to sleep with the pillow behind you, within grasping distance. Patients have told me that if they go to sleep this way, they reach for the pillow automatically during the night when they roll over on their side.

The following chapter, Relaxation techniques, teaches a simple method to help you reduce the effects of stress.

CHAPTER FIVE

RELAXATION TECHNIQUES

This chapter gives a brief outline of the nature of stress and our understanding of its effects on the body, and provides an easy-to-learn practical approach to cultivating a relaxed state. The method is described in conceptual terms, with a script of the kind of words one may use in this practice. You may wish to record this script on a cassette (or ask a friend with a soothing voice to record it for you) to play while you practise. The script contains a mental checklist of the important points to cover and includes guided visualisation techniques that can help overcome neck or back pain. The script can be adapted to any similar purpose, such as performance enhancement in sport. Details will be found at the end of this chapter.

Practical Stress Management seminars

Most of this chapter is drawn from the Practical Stress Management seminars I do for private companies and senior and middle management levels of government. Usually slotted into the middle of a week of workshops devoted to more conventional management techniques, these seminars have been received extremely well. In them, I use a number of the most important exercises presented in this book to show each manager precisely (and dramatically) where he or she actually holds tension resulting from daily stress. The whole seminar lasts two and a half hours, but in this chapter I present a slightly more formal version of the last thirty minutes, which teaches a quick way of learning how to relax. Do not be put off by my use of the word 'quick'. The method combines elements of old and new techniques, and is more effective than any single approach I have come across to date. It is now accepted that one's mental state can be altered by changing one's physical state, and the converse is also true. To this point in the book, we have dealt with the physical almost exclusively, but it is now time to consider the mental–physical nexus.

In passing, it may be useful to contrast the attitudes of the participants of these courses with those of our students in the *Posture & Flexibility* classes. Whether a defence against appearing vulnerable in front of their peers or whether a function of a typical mix of personality traits displayed by managers, the suggestion that learning how to relax will be directly useful is usually met with scepticism, especially by the male participants. Evidently, most managers believe (or affect the belief when they are in these groups) that non-mainstream medicine or practices are somehow strange or weird. I am usually greeted by a sea of raised eyebrows, folded arms and similar body language when I first enter the seminar room—a tough audience, in other words.

When I began giving these seminars, I used to mount what I considered to be unassailable arguments, supported by evidence drawn from different areas of research, and all converging on the position I was advocating. With an academic audience, this strategy may have succeeded, but it failed completely with the more pragmatic managers. Accordingly, I gave thought to how one might quickly and thoroughly convince an audience of the worth of the ideas and techniques presented.

I decided to use a neck exercise as a demonstration in the first minutes of the presentation. I use the sitting side stretch for the neck, complete with the contraction and relaxation parts. All participants' necks move closer to the shoulder after doing this, and I then ask them to repeat for the other side, comparing left with right. By this time (two minutes later) audience attention and participation is always 100%. The old adage that you can take a horse to water but you cannot make it drink is true, as far as it goes. A different approach is to make that horse *feel* thirsty. I use this approach with relaxation techniques I teach as the concluding part of these seminars. I offer no explanation at all, and go directly to the script (at the end of this chapter), so the participants can *feel* the value of the techniques. Here though, before we get to the script I shall present a brief discussion of the whys and wherefores of relaxation.

Why relax?

Stress is a much-used and abused term in the languages of medicine and 'human resource management'. Originally an engineering term, it was brought into medicine by the pioneer of this research, Dr Hans Selye. Selye conceived of stress as those aspects of the environment that provoke a response in the organism. He divided stress into *eustress*, or good stress, and *distress*, which includes the familiar meaning. The originality of Selye's research lies mainly in his elucidation of the physical processes that mediate these stresses— the adrenal glands and their associated hormones—and his demonstration that the two types of stress (perceived so differently by the individual) have remarkably similar physiological effects on the body.

The effects of stress have been labelled as the 'fight or flight' response. They are characterised by physical and psychological changes such as increased respiration and pulse rates, increased blood pressure, increased sympathetic nervous system activity, and increased feelings of 'pressure'. Physiologists assume that these responses prepare the organism (for these responses are not limited to humans) for fighting or evading danger in the environment. Further, they assume that modern humans are the result of past evolutionary forces, and hence very likely to be the progeny of organisms who were successful in coping with these kinds of pressures. However, these responses may well be inappropriate in the modern office environment. This change to our normal environment is the crux of Selye's research. If one does not fight or flee, the crucial question is what happens to the body if this response (with all its accompanying hormones, increased blood sugar and other metabolic changes) is repeatedly activated and not used?

Without doubt, one common result is the disease known as the 'silent killer'— hypertension, or permanently elevated blood pressure. This condition is considered to be a major predisposing cause of many fatal heart conditions and similar serious diseases. Everyone is aware of the momentary muscular effects of being frightened or angry (immediately increased tension in all the muscles of the body). However, the main effect of the *repeated* activation of this response is permanently elevated tension in the muscles of the body. Elevated muscle tension may even be the primary cause of hypertension. Either way, those muscles that are 'pre-stressed' for one reason or another are precisely those muscles of concern to us here—the neck and back muscles. I believe that our evolutionary inheritance, coupled with a sedentary lifestyle, is the main reason neck and back pain is so commonplace.

Fortunately, there is a complementary physiological and psychological response, tentatively named the 'relaxation response' (Benson, 1976), which can be cultivated simply by everyone. This response appears to be controlled by the *hypothalamus,* just as the fight or flight response is. The effects of the relaxation response are the opposite of those of the fight or flight response, and also include the effect of reduced tension in the muscles of the body. It is not at all clear why most people are more effective at mobilising the fight or flight response rather than the relaxation response, but I suspect that evolutionary pressures favoured the former and not the latter. The relaxation response—which everyone demonstrates to some degree—can be vastly enhanced and actively used to counter the stress of life.

For the sufferer of neck or back pain, learning how to access this response may be used in the short term to cope with the pain or discomfort of an attack (by making the relevant muscles relax). It can also be used in the medium to long term to increase the 'headroom' between the normal state of the muscles and the kind of tension which predisposes one to an attack. Together with the stretching and strengthening exercises, improving the relaxation response forms a highly efficient multi-stranded approach to alleviating the problem.

Relaxation method

I shall use Benson's four elements leading to 'the elicitation of the Relaxation Response' (p.78 ff.) to structure my recommendations for your practice. In passing, it should be noted that Benson's book outlines the major research done in various techniques said to lead to a relaxed or meditative state. He found that all the disciplines considered—regardless of cultural origin—shared many common methods and resulted in virtually identical physiological states. For an excellent and not-too-technical review, I recommend this book for further reading on this fascinating subject.

The first requirement, according to Benson, is a quiet environment in which to do one's practice. Although a quiet place is useful to learn how to feel this relaxation response (and then how to create it at will), it is not essential later (for example, it is commonplace in Japan for people to meditate on trains, very noisy places indeed). An interesting aspect of this relaxed state (and one of the ways you will know you have achieved it) is that, although sounds around you seem further away, you can still attend to their essential content, but in a rather more detached way than usual. In normal daily life, you should find a time and a place where you are not likely to be disturbed. Before dinner or before sleep are especially good times for many people. And for the reasons given earlier, it is best to seclude yourself from your spouse and children. A three-year-old child regards the prone body as a direct invitation to crawl and play, and this will not help your practice! Similarly, pull the 'phone out of the wall. You will need only ten to fifteen minutes of peace and quiet.

Benson's second element is 'a mental device', like repeating a sound to yourself, concentrating your gaze on a symbol, or concentrating on a feeling. The last recommendation I have found to be the most effective, and I shall expand on this point below.

The third element is 'a passive attitude', an 'emptying of all thoughts and distractions from one's mind' (p.78). I spent a long time in Zen temples in Japan trying to do just this little thing. As any of you who have tried to do this will know, it is *extremely* hard to do (it is like someone saying to you 'whatever you think of, don't think about pink elephants!'). Being able to 'empty your mind' is the mark of an adept, and not the best approach for beginners who need another approach—in effect, something appropriate to fill the mind.

Benson's last element is 'a comfortable position'. Various sitting positions are the recommendations of both Zen and yoga, although some sects' practitioners meditate while walking. Lying down is usually not recommended, because in the untrained individual it often leads to sleep. We are trying to find that mental and physical state where we seem to be hovering between wakefulness and sleep, and falling asleep is not desirable. In my experience, it is perfectly possible to meditate in any comfortable position. The recommendations about sitting in the lotus pose, for example, are completely inappropriate for all but yoga practitioners. Until you can sit in this pose in perfect comfort for ten or fifteen minutes, the sensations in your legs are guaranteed to distract you from the purpose, deep relaxation. However, if you *can* sit in this pose for the required time, it is ideal because it locks the hips and enables you to keep a straight back without effort.

My recommendations for practice are to lie stretched out face-up on the floor without a pillow, providing this is comfortable. The floor is better than a bed, because you do not want to drift off to sleep, and the associations will be difficult for the mind and the body to ignore. If your back is sore, or if lying on the floor with the legs stretched out is uncomfortable, put a pillow or similar object under the knees to flex the legs. This will not detract from the effect we are seeking. Wear warm clothing or cover yourself with a blanket. Loosen any tight clothing, particularly collars and belts. Make sure that you do not need to go to the toilet in the next 15 minutes.

Place one hand flat on your chest and the other flat on your abdomen, above the navel. Many people do not breathe abdominally but breathe mostly into the top of the chest. Most physiologists believe that chest breathing is not optimally efficient, because it requires the 'muscles of inspiration' to be used in addition to the diaphragm. These neck, shoulder and rib muscles are used together with the diaphragm when we are breathing really deeply (for example, when you sprint for the bus or as you sit gasping in the bus recovering from the unaccustomed run). However, these muscles are not the ones to use when learning how to relax. For this reason, when you begin practice, place your hands as suggested. As you breathe in, you will feel the hand over the navel rise as the abdomen is pressed out by the diaphragm contracting. Ideally, the hand on the chest should not move. If it does, try to feel how to breathe so that it does not. Once you feel the difference, practice will be easy. Imagine the breath flowing deep into the abdomen while you try to feel it. Like many things, it is more a matter of awareness than the need to develop a special skill.

I do not share the common recommendation of having an object to dwell on or a sound (mantra) to chant. Of course, if you already practise this way successfully, please continue to do so. Obviously, a beginner will find it helpful to concentrate on *something*, and in place of an object or sound, I suggest you divide your concentration between two aspects of your practice, changing from one to the other as distracting thoughts occur. In this way, you will be able to combine two of Benson's elements in a new way to produce the desired effect.

To begin, lie as suggested and close your eyes. You may like to have soothing music on in the background, especially something repetitive and structured without dramatic passages. If you have recorded the script I suggest below, you can play it, either on headphones or on a stereo. Alternatively, you could record it with suitable music playing in the background. Concentrate on one part of the body, starting with the feet, in turn. Determine whether that part feels comfortable. If it does not, or if you are not sure whether it is as relaxed as it could be, make a small movement to bring the toes closer to each other and relax, letting the feet fall outwards. (In this case, the position of the feet is controlled by the hip muscles, but because the action of the hip joint produces movement of the feet, it is convenient to think of it as a foot movement.)

Next consider for a moment the sensation of how the foot position feels. The concentration is then shifted to the breath. Breathe in and out three times, not making any effort to control the breathing (that is, make no effort to slow or deepen the breathing). Here, we adopt a passive attitude of 'seeing' the breath come into, and leave, the body. Concentrate on the many sensations accompanying this most familiar of activities, but of which we usually are completely unaware—the feeling of air flowing through the nose and down the throat, and so on. Feel the rise and fall of the abdomen. Following the three breaths, return your concentration to the body, to the next part in the sequence presented in the script. From this we return to the breath, each time using a slightly different way of breathing, which I explain in the script.

In this way, we are dividing the concentration between two distinct sets of feelings, each rich with sensation. Such concentration fills the brain with information—and hence stops the thoughts that normally rush into one's mind in the absence of thought. This is my way of emptying the mind. It is an active way of avoiding the normal distractions, and leads you into a relaxed state effortlessly and without frustration. The concentration span required in each breath phase is deliberately brief. Teaching this technique has shown that a beginner cannot maintain concentration easily on even a five-breath cycle (of about twenty seconds). By swapping one's concentration relatively quickly between the two foci of attention, the mind does not have enough time to become bored or restless with any one set of thought. The experiences thus remain alive and consuming, with no space for distraction.

Guided visualisation and healing the body

A new field of research in western medicine (not much more than ten years old) is called *psychoneuroimmunology* (psycho-neuro-immunology). It attempts to uncover the processes and relationships between psychological and physiological states. This research has revealed many mechanisms underlying our common-sense knowledge of how the world works, including the vitally important links between mood (mental state) and function (physiological process). The research strongly supports the claim (made by many alternative health practitioners) that healing processes can be aided by thinking or feeling them into a more powerful response. I have included an excellent overview of this research as suggested further reading, a book called *Imagery in Healing*. Visualisation of certain healing processes, when one is in an appropriately relaxed state, can speed the process. Similar visualisation can be used to reduce the sensation of chronic pain or for other purposes. Accordingly, I have included a brief mention of useful visualisations for neck or back pain. A little imagination will allow you to adapt this script for other kinds of pain or to enhance performance of particular skills. Research has shown that this visualisation fires the neurons involved (but at a sub-maximal level, so little movement of the involved muscles occurs), effectively rehearsing the skill without actually doing it. You may wish to expand this pain control section before you have the script recorded, adding specific details relevant to your situation.

Before we begin, let me remind you of the important check points—go to the toilet, take the 'phone off the hook, loosen any tight clothing and put on warm clothing.

A script for relaxation and visualisation

(A note to the person recording the script: allow three to five seconds pause between paragraphs as marked. Speak in a normal, but unhurried voice, without dramatic changes in intonation or pitch. Try to stay relaxed yourself as you record the script, and resist the common temptation to hurry your delivery.)

Lie down on a firm surface and close your eyes. We are going on a journey around the body, a journey designed to take you into a state of deep relaxation.

We'll begin with the feet. Adjust their position, using the smallest movements that will have the desired effect. Bring the toes together a fraction, and let the feet fall to the sides. Wriggle the toes of the left foot a little until the foot feels completely comfortable. Now the right foot. Arch the foot and let it relax. Move the toes a little. Now try to feel both feet at the same time. Feel the weight of the feet press down onto the floor through the heels. Make sure that the heels feel comfortable.

Now, turn your attention to the breath. Begin by taking three relaxed breaths in and out. Don't try to slow or deepen your breathing. See and feel how the breath moves in and out of the body of its own accord. It is rhythmic and tidal. Feel the air move through the nose. See it going down the throat into the lungs. Feel it lifting the abdomen under your hand. Feel how the breath flows, in and out.

Back to the body. Start with the right leg this time. Feel how the leg is resting on the floor, through the calf muscle. Often, this muscle is not as relaxed as it can be. To make sure, gently bring the toes of the right foot a small distance towards the right knee. Then let the foot relax to its most comfortable position. Now the left foot. Move the toes a little in the direction of the left knee, and let the left foot go. Feel the weight of both legs at the same time. You can feel their weight pressing onto the floor. Both legs feel relaxed, the heels and calf muscles resting comfortably on the floor.

For this next series of breaths, hold the breath *in* for a count of two. Keep the throat open, and hold the breath in by using just the diaphragm to keep the abdomen open for a count of two. Breathe in, and hold—one, two. Now let the breath go out without forcing it in any way. See and feel the breath leaving the body. Repeat this cycle two more times. Breathe in. Hold—one, two. Let the breath go. Breathe in. Hold—one two. Let the breath go.

Turn your attention back to the body. From the legs, the next part of the body to contact the floor is the bottom. Make sure that the bottom is resting on the floor as comfortably as it can. Briefly and gently tighten the bottom muscles. Then let the muscles go completely soft. Now feel the weight of the bottom on the floor. Feel the weight of the whole of the legs, from the heels through the calf muscles to the bottom. This part of the body feels heavy now. As you become more relaxed it is normal for your body to feel heavier and heavier. It is a pleasant feeling. You are starting to feel somewhat detached from your surroundings, aware but a little distant.

This time, hold the breath *out* for a count of two. Hold the breath out by using the abdominal muscles. Keep the throat open. Breathe in normally. Don't hold the breath in this time. As soon as the lungs are full, breathe out. At the end of the breath out, breathe out a little more forcefully than before. Feel the stomach muscles tighten as you breathe out. Hold the breath out, and count—one, two. Relax, and let the air rush in. Feel its movement fill the lungs. Repeat this cycle two more times in your own time. [If you are recording this script, pause for enough time for the next two breath cycles to be completed.]

Turn your attention back to the body. The next part of the body to contact the floor is the back and the shoulders. Begin with the left shoulder. Very gently take its weight off the floor. Let it rest on the floor again. Now the right shoulder. Does it feel completely relaxed? If not, move it a small amount until it does. Does the part of your back on the floor feel completely comfortable? If not, move a small amount from side to side until it does. Now feel the weight of the whole body on the floor. You become aware of the weight of your body as you become more relaxed. It is a wonderful feeling of stillness, of being relaxed, of being comfortable.

This time, hold the breath both in *and* out. Breathe in. Hold the breath in for a count of one, two. Let the breath go out now. Feel the air going out of the body. At the end, breathe out the last part. Hold the breath out—one, two. In your own time, repeat this two more times. Do not force the breathing in or out. Do not try too hard. Relax with each breath out.

And now to the last part of the body, the head. Move the head a little from side to side to relax the neck muscles. Do they feel completely comfortable? You may need to tilt the head back a little, or it may need to come forward to feel completely comfortable on the floor. Now feel the enormous weight of the whole body, pressing on the floor from heels, calf muscles, through the bottom, the back and shoulders, and the head. Feel the body as one thing, pressing onto the floor. The body feels relaxed now, and it feels good. See yourself lying on the floor from above. You look completely relaxed.

Back to the breathing. This time, make no effort of any kind at all. Visualise the breath coming into the body. See it as a colour. Choose one you like. Which colour doesn't matter. See the breath coming in through the nose, going down the throat, and into the lungs. Feel it going into the lungs. Feel the tummy rise. As you breathe out, imagine the breath as a different colour. Feel any tension remaining in the body going out with the breath. That's why it's now a different colour. The more vividly you can visualise this, the more effective it will become. For the next cycle, concentrate your whole attention on five breaths in and out. If you find your attention wandering, turn it back to the body. If you are recording this script, pause long enough for four or five more breath cycles.

And now back to the body. Feel the weight of the head on the floor again. Check to see whether the jaw muscles are holding tension. If you are not sure, lightly clench the teeth and let these muscles relax fully. Feel the muscles in the cheeks. Are they holding any tension? If so, lightly purse the lips, and let the face relax. Now the forehead. Frown briefly. Raise the eyebrows. Then let all the muscles of the face rest in their most relaxed positions. The face is a relaxed mask, now. It is serene. Feel the weight of the whole body now. It is pressing on the floor. It feels very heavy. It feels completely relaxed and comfortable. Feel this complex of sensations. This is what being relaxed feels like. It feels wonderful. You may feel as though you are floating. Or you may feel as though you are somehow removed from your surroundings. Sounds around you seem further away, and although you can still hear everything, the sounds do not disturb you.

Feel your breathing now. Imagine small waves breaking on a quiet beach. A little wave comes in, it lifts itself up, and breaks on the shore. As the water recedes, it makes a long hissing sound. It is a relaxing sound. It is a timeless sound. The movement of the waves is ceaseless. Your breath comes in as a little wave picks itself up. It goes out as the water recedes. Each breath out sounds like the water going out. Hear the sounds of the beach around you. Hear the faint cries of the gulls, the sounds of the water. Feel a soft breeze on your face. You feel at peace with the world. Your body feels relaxed and heavy. You feel safe and secure. Concentrate on a few breaths, in and out.

This is the state of deep relaxation. You feel completely comfortable. Your body is healing itself as you relax in this state. The tension in your muscles is leaving the body with every breath out. It is now time to direct the healing processes to where they are needed. See your sore spots in your mind. Direct a healing flow of energy to these places. Imagine a coloured light bathing these places. Imagine your body's healing processes at work. The more vividly you can see these things happening inside your body, the more effective they will be.

If you are recording this script, pause for about thirty seconds. If you wish to adapt the script for sporting or skill performance, this is the place to insert the relevant cues. For example, if you wish to mentally rehearse a skill such as shooting baskets or putting, have the person recording the script say (for example) 'Now see yourself shooting 20 baskets, perfectly'. Mention in particular the aspects you wish to improve in as much detail as you can—the more detail, the better.

Your neck and back feel better than before, and you are going to feel better still as time goes on. Knots in your muscles are being smoothed away as tension leaves your body. The muscles of your neck and back feel more relaxed than they've ever been. These muscles feel warm, now. They feel comfortable, relaxed, and good. You know that tension prevents the body from healing itself. You are going to try to release tension from the body with each breath out, in your normal daily life.

Tell yourself it's good to be relaxed. It feels good to be relaxed. The stresses and strains of life do not affect me, now. And each time I practise, I improve. The state of deep relaxation comes to me faster than the last time I practised, and the state of relaxation deeper as I practise. Each breath out relaxes you that tiny bit more. You are on a path which leads you to feeling more and more relaxed. Feel the feeling of deep relaxation. If you are recording this script, leave a long pause here—a minute or two.

Now you want to rouse yourself from your deeply relaxed state. Some of the effects of deep relaxation will stay with you when you are fully awake. To come back to the normal world, breathe in deeply. Fill the whole of the chest. At the same time, raise your arms straight up and stretch them out behind you, back onto the floor. Press your toes away from you. Stretch your entire body. Breathe out as you bring your arms back to your sides. Stretch them out again, and breathe in fully. Bring the arms back to your sides, and relax. Sit up when you are ready. Note: this script's available in a recorded form on cassette, called *The Relaxation Script*.

REFERENCES

Bolton, S. P., 1987. Similarities and differences between Chiropractic and Osteopathy. *J. Aust. Chiropr. Assoc.*, 17: 90–93.

Bradbeer, M., 1985. Nursing back from stress. *Forceps*, Mar.: 71–72.

Brooks, P. M., 1987. Back pain in the workplace. *Med. J. Aust.*, 147: 257–258.

Charlton, K. H., 1988. Approaches to the demonstration of vertebral subluxation: 1. Introduction and manual diagnosis: A review. *J. Aust. Chiropr. Assoc.*, 18: 9–13.

Ganora, A., 1984. Chronic back pain: diagnosis, treatment and rehabilitation. *Patient Management*, Aug.: 55–79.

Giles, L. G. F. and Taylor, J. R., 1985. Low-back pain associated with leg-length inequality. *J. Aust. Chiropr. Assoc.*, 15: 135–145.

Heere, L., 1986. The spine in sports. *N.Z. J. Sports Med.*, Dec. : 90–92.

Henderson, I., 1985. Low back pain and sciatica: evaluation and surgical management. *Australian Family Physician*, 14: 1149–1159.

Hoppenfeld, S., 1976. *Physical examination of the spine and extremities.* Prentice-Hall International, Inc., Englewood Cliffs, New Jersey.

Jensen, M. C., Brant-Zawadski, M. N., Obuchowski, N., Modic, M.T., Malkasian, D., and Ross, J. S., 1994. Magnetic resonance imaging of the lumbar spine in people without back pain. *New England Journal of Medicine*, July 14. 331, No. 2: 69–73.

Kapandji, I. A., 1974. *The Physiology of the Joints.* Volume Three. Churchill Livingstone, Edinburgh.

Kendall, H.O., Kendall, F.P., and Wadsworth, G.P., 1971. *Muscles, Testing and Function.* 2nd edition. Williams and Wilkins, Baltimore.

Knott, M., and Voss, D.E., 1968. *Proprioceptive Neuromuscular Facilitation.* Harper & Row, New York.

Kolata, G., 1994. Study raises serious doubts about commonly used methods of treating back pain. *New York Times*, July 14, 1994, p. A9 (California edition).

Laughlin, K., 1989. Low back pain: review and prescription. In *Is our future limited by our past?* Freeman, L. (ed.). Proceedings of the third conference of the Australasian Society for Human Biology. The Australasian Society for Human Biology, University of Western Australia.

Littler, T. R., 1983. Low back pain. *Update*, May: 59–73.

Macquarie, 1981. *The Macquarie Dictionary,* 2nd edition, revised 1987.

Murtagh, J., 1983. Examination and diagnosis of low backache. *Australian Family Physician*, 12: 322–328.

Murtagh, J., Findlay, D., and Kenna, C., 1985. Low back pain. *Australian Family Physician*, 14: 1214–1224.

Porkert, M., 1974. *The Theoretical Foundations of Chinese Medicine: systems of correspondence.* MIT Press, Cambridge.

Rock, B. A., 1988. Short leg—a review and survey. *J. Aust. Chiropr. Assoc.*, 18: 91–96.

Saal, J. A., 1988. Rehabilitation of football players with lumbar spine injury (part 1 of 2). *The Physician and Sportsmedicine*, 16: 61–68.

Travell, J.G. and Simons, D.G., Volume 1, 1983; Volume 2, 1992. *Myofascial Pain and Dysfunction: The Trigger Point Manual.* Williams & Wilkins, Baltimore.

Twomey, L. T., 1974. Low back pain. Proceedings of a conference on low back pain held at the W.A.I.T. Bentley Campus, Sept. 14–15. School of Health Sciences, Western Australia Institute of Technology.

Wells, K. F. and Luttgens, K.,1976. *Kinesiology: Scientific Basis of Human Motion*, 6th edition. Saunders College, Philadelphia.

FURTHER READING

Achterberg, J., 1985. *Imagery in healing: shamanism and modern medicine.* New Science Library, Boston and London.

Benson, H., 1976. *The Relaxation Response.* Collins, London.

ACKNOWLEDGMENTS

The writing of a book may be undertaken lightly, but if my experience is anything to go by, seldom will it be finished the same way. And so it was with this book—I am glad that I could not know how much sheer work it would take. Many people have helped and encouraged me along the way.

My primary debt of gratitude goes to my business partner, Paul Bottari. (By way of aside, I am irked by how one must attach a word like 'business' to the once perfectly adequate word 'partner', with its nuance of a mutually advantageous contract.) It is conventional to say things like 'without his help, this book could not have been written'. In this case, saying so would be inadequate. Paul provided me with financial support and friendship at many stages up to the final draft, and through to production and distribution. I am deeply grateful.

Although mentioned in the text, I wish to thank again the teachers of *Posture & Flexibility*, Carol Wenzel, David Moten (travelling around the world, somewhere), my brother Dr Greg Laughlin, Mark Donohue, Jennifer Cristaudo, and Petra Boevink. Unfailingly cheerful and dedicated teachers, all. One or two might even be described as over-enthusiastic. I make a special thank you to Jennifer, who modelled for the pictures and commented on an early draft. Thank you, Greg, for reading a draft (making suggestions which separated the strands of the argument far more clearly), and for making life interesting (we share a house).

Kathy Sharpe (what a name for a photographer) came from Sydney to Canberra a number of times to take the photographs, for a miserly remuneration. Next book at full professional rates, Kathy, I promise. Kathy did the darkroom work, too.

When I received the manuscript back from editor Dr Michael Nunn, I could hardly see the words for the overlay of purple ink. However, after sober consideration of his liberal wielding of the purple pen (including some painful excisions), there was no doubt that the argument flowed better and the usages were more consistent. Thank you for the effort you put in. Any faults in the text remain mine alone, of course.

I appreciate the assistance given by the Zoo Illustrative Group here in Canberra   Jeremy Mears designed the cover and manipulated the images and photographs (all digitally), Zoë D'Arcy did the book design and layout, Catherine Eadie did the illustrations and Cameron (the Zoo keeper) supervised. Mrs Mears' cats kept both Jeremy and I amused during this period. Typos are the cats' responsibility.

Traditional practitioners of medicine have said that one receives the best care from someone who has suffered what ails you. I hope that this is true—but in addition to my experiences, I wish to acknowledge the invaluable contributions of both my patients and the students in the classes. As Alfred E. Neuman (*Mad Magazine*) once said, 'You may as well learn from everyone else's mistakes; you're not going to live long enough to make them all yourself'— I have learned virtually everything I know about neck and back pain from working with these groups.

Last, I wish to thank Megan and Ted for their respective special contributions.

AFTERWORD TO THE SECOND EDITION

It is now a year since the release of the first edition of *Overcome neck & back pain*, and it seems fitting that I reflect on the book's passage, and the events leading to the publishing of the revised second edition by Simon & Schuster. After we had sold 4000 copies of the first edition, I sent copies to the three publishers who, almost exactly one year previously, had rejected the manuscript, asking them for assistance in overseas distribution. Two days later, the managing director of Simon & Schuster, Jon Attenborough, called me; we set up a meeting for the next week, and shook hands on an arrangement the same day. In the ordinary way of these things of course, the contracts took rather longer to finalise... I want to express my appreciation to Jon Attenborough and Lynne Segal for their help in facilitating this edition, and I look forward to a long association.

I have had enormous feedback from the first edition, from readers, practitioners of all persuasions, colleagues at the Australian National University, and friends. The list of illustrations and the Quick Reference in particular are a result of these suggestions. I have been gratified particularly by all those who wrote to me telling me of their experiences with the exercises. Many people took the trouble to come to the Shoshin Centre from interstate, and I have worked with a number of professional athletes and musicians with good results. Using exercises as a treatment protocol requires feeding the user's impressions and reactions back into the approach, and the additions and modifications to the exercises presented here reflect a year's work of this sort: more C–R stretches and additional variations to the standard versions of the exercises.

On a personal note, I wish to acknowledge my intellectual debt to Dr Richard Sylvan, who died this year. He was an inspiration to me, and chapter four partly grew out of my fascination with his relevant logic and his fearlessness in crossing traditional disciplinary boundaries. He built houses in addition to systems of logic, and his insistence that particular systems needed tying to the real world resonates in me still.

I wish to thank Jeremy again for his work in manipulating the bits and bytes comprising the second edition of this book. *Overcome neck & back pain* is still one of the few books that has been digitally constructed in its entirety, including all illustrations, photographs, text, and the cover, which made all the changes considerably less burdensome than they would have been otherwise. My thanks to Julia Topliss, who shot the additional photographs.

The team of *Posture & Flexibility* teachers has grown by three: Olivia Allnutt, an ex-gymnast, Matt Baker, an ex-member of the Canberra *Raiders* squad, and Pierre Le Count, *Posture & Flexibility*'s hardest working student. With *Strength & Flexibility*, we now teach more than 20 classes per week at the Australian National University Sports Union. My thanks again to this intrepid band, all of whom have done so much to improve the method as presented here.

While most of you were having holidays over Christmas last year, we made two complementary video tapes: *Overcome neck, arm & shoulder pain* and *Overcome back pain*. The former has all the neck exercises from the book, plus all the arm, forearm, shoulder and hand exercises we use in the clinic and the classes, as we have found that few people who have neck pain do not have problems in these other areas too. The latter has all the back exercises (including the new hip exercise, 36) and the two most important strengthening exercises. Both video tapes are about an hour long. I have recorded *The relaxation script* (chapter five) on audio cassette also; it is twenty minutes long. All are available from selected stores or from us directly on **1-800-800-590.**

QUICK REFERENCE